Unifying Nursing Languages

The Harmonization of NANDA, NIC, and NOC

Joanne McCloskey Dochterman, PhD, RN, FAAN
and Dorothy A. Jones, EdD, RNC, FAAN
Editors

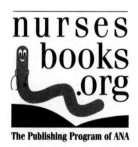

nurses
books
.org

The Publishing Program of ANA

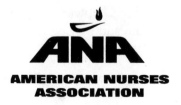

ANA

AMERICAN NURSES
ASSOCIATION

WASHINGTON, D.C.

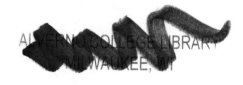

Library of Congress Cataloging-in-Publication Data

Unifying nursing languages : the harmonization of NANDA, NIC, and NOC /
Joanne McCloskey Dochterman and Dorothy Jones, editors.
      p. ; cm.
Includes bibliographical references.
  ISBN 1-55810-208-6
  1. Nursing—Classification.
  [DNLM: 1. Nursing. 2. Vocabulary, Controlled. Z 695.1.N8 U58 2003]
I. Dochterman, Joanne McCloskey. II. Jones, Dorothy A.

RT42U554 2003
610.73′01′2—dc21

                              2003004483

Published by
NursesBooks.org
600 Maryland Avenue, SW
Suite 100 West
Washington, D.C. 20024-2571

ISBN 1-55810-208-6

UNL23   1.5M   03/03

Contents

Preface and Invitation

This monograph presents the process, content, and outcomes of the project funded by a National Library of Medicine grant (R13 LMO7243). The grant supported an invitational conference with a three-fold focus: articulating the assumptions underlying the individual languages of diagnoses, interventions, and outcomes; examining the existing taxonomic structures; and identifying the issues and preparing a first draft of a common taxonomic structure. The conference brought together leaders in nursing language development to create a common unifying structure across the three classification systems: NANDA for nursing diagnoses, NIC for nursing interventions, and NOC for nursing outcomes. You hold the results of that conference in your hands.

The editors, who were awarded the grant, serve as co-chairs of the NNN Alliance. The NNN Alliance represents a virtual and collaborative relationship between the North American Nursing Diagnosis Association (NANDA) and the Center for Nursing Classification and Clinical Effectiveness (CNC) at the University of Iowa. This alliance was created to advance the development, testing, and refinement of nursing language.

Having a common structure is more efficient than having separate structures and facilitates implementation of all the languages in practice and education. Many groups stand to benefit from a common unified nursing language classification, including educators, clinicians, researchers, and administrators. As well, informatics specialists will be able to integrate a common unified classification of nursing language into their development of information systems that can benefit from refinement, accuracy, and clarity of terms used to communicate nursing to others.

The contents of this monograph, however important a step forward for nursing science, are but a beginning. To advance nursing language overall and to increase its use throughout the discipline, continued feedback from all nurses will be needed. Since the common unifying structure proposed in these pages is in the public domain, nurses—whether involved in language development, education, administration and leadership, or clinical practice—are encouraged to use the classification and help in its refinement. Opportunities to discuss the strengths and limitations of the proposed common structure will arise at open nursing forums, on web sites (www.nanda.org or www.nursing.uiowa.edu/cnc), and at the next NNN conference, to be held in April 2004.

About the Authors

Joanne McCloskey Dochterman, PhD, RN, Distinguished Professor and Director of the Center for Nursing at the University of Iowa College of Nursing, is co-Principal Investigator (with Gloria Bulechek) of the Nursing Interventions Classification (NIC). She is a past member of the NANDA Board of Directors and co-chair of the NNN Alliance. She has also participated in the national efforts to develop a Reference Terminology Model for nursing. She has an extensive research and funding background in the areas of nursing administration and classification. She has participated in various efforts to link NIC and NOC with NANDA.

Dorothy A. Jones, EdD, RNC,FAAN, Professor, Boston College, Boston, MA is the immediate Past President of NANDA; she serves as Co-Chair of the NNN Alliance. She brings her work in knowledge development, nursing informatics and language development to this project. Dr. Jones has conducted multiple funded research projects that helped to identify nursing phenomena (interventions and outcomes) within a variety of clinical populations. In addition, she has developed and established the psychometric properties of the Functional Health Pattern Assessment Screening Tool (FHPAST), which uses as a conceptual framework the work of Gordon (1994). Dr. Jones has authored numerous publications in the area of nursing language.

Geoffrey C. Bowker, PhD, Professor in the Department of Communication at the University of San Diego, La Jolla, California. He has spent his academic career studying the structure of knowledge in various disciplines. He presented the keynote talk on the science of classification at the NNN 2001 conference and assisted in laying important groundwork for collaboration.

Margaret Lunney, PhD, RN, Professor and Program Coordinator, Master of Science in Adult Health Nursing at the College of Staten Island, City University of New York, has long involvement in NANDA and numerous publications on nursing diagnosis and critical thinking. Dr. Lunney completed an NIH funded study of the effects of using NANDA, NIC, and NOC on the health outcomes of school children. Her clinical and teaching background is in adult health and community health.

Introduction: The Groundwork for Unification 1

*Joanne McCloskey Dochterman
and Dorothy Jones*

In 1973, Kristine Gebbie and Mary Ann Lavin held the First Conference on the Classification of Nursing Diagnoses, a conference designed to classify health problems within the domain of nursing (Gebbie & Lavin 1975). This group later became known as the North American Nursing Diagnosis Association (NANDA). Over the years, other classifications, including the Nursing Interventions Classification (NIC) and the Nursing Outcomes Classification (NOC), were developed. As NANDA, NIC, and NOC have grown, each group has worked independently to classify, name, and define diagnoses, interventions, and outcomes in three separate structures. In an effort to promote the consistent use of a unified disciplinary language by all nurses, NANDA and the Center for Nursing Classification and Clinical Effectiveness at the University of Iowa (home to NIC and NOC) created a virtual NNN Alliance to facilitate movement toward the development of a unified nursing classification.

NANDA, NIC, and NOC: The NNN Alliance

The NNN Alliance represents a virtual and collaborative relationship between the North American Nursing Diagnosis Association (NANDA) and the Center for Nursing Classification and Clinical Effectiveness (CNC) at the University of Iowa College of Nursing. The goal of this alliance is to advance the development, testing, and refinement of nursing language. This goal has been realized in part through the development of a grant proposal, designed to bring together leaders in nursing language development in order to create a common unifying structure across the three classification systems (i.e., NANDA—nursing diagnoses, NIC—nursing interventions, and NOC—nursing outcomes).

In 2001, Joanne Dochterman and Dorothy A. Jones, co-chairs of the NNN Alliance, received a grant from the National Library of Medicine (R13 LMO7243). The purpose of the grant was to support an invitational conference to focus on:

▮ articulating the assumptions underlying each language (diagnoses, interventions, and outcomes);

■ examining existing taxonomic structures; and

■ identifying issues and preparing a first draft of a common taxonomic structure.

Nursing leaders involved in nursing language classifications—particularly nursing diagnoses (North American Nursing Diagnosis Association, NANDA), nursing interventions (Nursing Interventions Classification, NIC) and nursing outcomes (Nursing Outcomes Classification, NOC)—were invited to participate in the conference.

Invitational Conference

In August 2001, an invitational conference was held at the Starved Rock Conference Center in Utica, Illinois, during which the participants studied existing language classifications, nomenclatures, and data sets. At the completion of the conference, a small task force compiled the work of the conference attendees and created the first draft of a common unifying structure for diagnoses, interventions, and outcomes (NANDA, NIC, and NOC). The proposed structure was then disseminated among conference participants and exposed to the nursing community for feedback at the NNN Alliance International Conference in April 2002 and on the NANDA and CNC web sites.

Feedback from nurse colleagues was on a international level, and revisions to the document were made on the basis of this new information. The manuscript, entitled *Collaboration in Nursing Classification: The Creation of a Common Unifying Structure for NANDA, NIC and NOC*, was prepared by Dochterman and Jones and is the second chapter in the present monograph. Table 2-6 (see Chapter 2, page 20) contains the proposed common structure. It is hoped that nurses interested in documentation, knowledge development, nursing classification, and language development, as well as information systems developers, educators, and administrators, will review and critique this document. This feedback will enable further refinement and testing of the proposed unifying structure.

Framework for Proposed Common Unifying Structure

The developers of the proposed common structure used the clinical reasoning process and problem solving along with the work of Donaldson and Crowley (1978) and the American Nurses Association's *Nursing's Social Policy Statement* (1995) to guide the creation of a unifying structure. This knowledge provided a framework that fostered the linkages among NANDA, NIC, and NOC classifications.

Nursing language developers have historically been concerned with classifying phenomena of concern to nursing. Changes that result from nursing interventions are measured and described by the achievement of outcomes. Problem solving and clinical reasoning have been used to process information about the patient experience. Problem solving is structured within a model that relies on data (cues) obtained through assessment, resulting in a judgment or the identification of a patient problem (diagnosis). Nursing's goal is to relieve the problem by linking the judgment and related data to interventions "that restore function, promote comfort and foster optimal health" (Jones 1997: 80). Outcomes are then measured, and responses to interventions are observed. Within nursing, the clinical reasoning process is guided by the ANA, according to *Standards of Clinical Nursing Practice, 2nd Edition.* (1998).

Donaldson and Crowley (1978) cited three core nursing principles that also informed the developers of the proposed common unifying structure. These principles include (a) concern with principles and laws that influence life principles, well-being, and optimum functioning of humans sick and well; (b) concern with the patterning of human behavior in interaction with the environment in critical life situations; and (c) concern with processes by which positive changes in health status are affected.

The American Nurses Association's *Nursing's Social Policy Statement* (1995) provided additional focus direction for developers. In particular, the *Social Policy Statement* states that "the phenomena of concern to nurses are human experiences and responses to birth, health, illness and death" (p. 8). The *Statement* goes on to define concepts that were central to the creation of the common structure, including (a) diagnoses, "the identification of responses to actual or potential health problems"; (b) interventions, "actions nurses take on behalf of patients and families or communities . . . to improve, correct or adjust physical, emotional, psychosocial, spiritual, cultural, and emotional conditions"; and (c) outcomes that evaluate "the effectiveness of interventions in relation to identified outcome" (pp. 1 & 9).

Knowledge from these resources provided the conference participants with a common framework to guide the creation of a unifying structure and to name and define domains and classes within the proposed classification. The framework was applicable to individuals, families, and communities and allowed for the integration of specific nursing theories to guide problem identification, diagnosis, intervention selection, and outcome evaluation.

Presentation Format for the Monograph

This monograph presents the process, content, and outcomes of the National Library of Medicine's funded project (Dochterman & Jones 2001). Conference papers and deliberations contained within the monograph are presented in three sections (1) the Main Paper, (2) Supporting Background Papers, and (3) Conclusion. In addition, three appendices are also incorporated into the document to support the presentations.

The Main Paper: Entitled "Collaboration in Nursing Classification: The Creation of a Common Unifying Structure for NANDA, NIC, and NOC," the main paper (Chapter 2) focuses on the invitational conference overall and on the iterative process for developing the common structure. The paper provides the background of existing nursing languages and the steps and methods used to generate a common unifying structure for NANDA, NIC, and NOC. The proposed common unifying structure for NNN includes domains and classes with definitions. The paper also discusses comments received since it was disseminated at the April 2002

NNN conference and web site responses; addresses issues concerning the overall structure, as well as term definitions and major unresolved issues; and reviews changes made in the structure since it was first developed.

Supporting Background Papers: The background papers include two papers presented during the Starved Rock Conference in order to provide the reader with additional information used by participants prior to developing the proposed common unifying structure.

The first paper is by Margaret Lunney, professor at the College of Staten Island, City University of New York. Her paper, entitled "Theoretical Explanations for Combining NANDA, NIC, and NOC," discusses the differences in the structures of NANDA, NIC, and NOC (NNN) and focuses on the difficulties users have encountered in identifying interrelationships among the three classification systems. The presentation speaks to past efforts to develop a common structure for NNN and their limitations related to practical utility without theoretical explanation. Lunney offers three theoretical explanations that support the significance of combining NNN: (1) Hayakawa's theory of linguistics, (2) critical thinking in nursing, and (3) the concept of accuracy and nursing diagnoses.

Hayakawa's theory of linguistics states that classification systems are essential for communication and collaboration and that the pooled knowledge within these systems helps us address the real world of nursing and practice. Critical thinking literature suggests that reducing the complexity of NNN will help improve the efficiency and effectiveness of nurses' discernment of diagnoses, interventions, and outcomes. Nursing diagnoses are more likely to be accurate when effective reasoning and critical thinking are associated with a more unified NNN.

Geoffrey Bowker, a professor in the Department of Communication at the University of California, San Diego, is the author of the second background paper, entitled "The Science and Art of Classification." Bowker addresses the central role of classification in both the scientific operation and organizational work of nursing and other professions. He also explores the strategy used by the August 2001 NNN invitational conference group in working with an interlocking set of classifications that focus on nursing work (nursing interventions), nursing diagnoses, and nursing outcomes. The paper draws on the literature in the study of classification in medicine, virology, and taxonomy to elucidate the features of nursing classification work. Bowker takes the example of the NIC classification, which he has studied over the past decade, to draw conclusions about the art of classification. The discussion supports the idea that classification work is central to the creation of professions and emphasizes that even though this work is often hidden from view, it is essential to the building of robust informational and organizational infrastructures.

Conclusion: Suggestions are made as to the uses of the proposed unifying nursing classification by educators, clinicians, researchers, and administrators.

Both NANDA and Mosby Year Book (the publisher of NIC and NOC) have given permission to include current labels and definitions in this monograph's appendices. As developers of NANDA, NIC, and NOC continue to expand or refine their existing classifications based upon research and clinical use, this information will appear in respective publications for each group. In the future, each group's publication will also include placement of NANDA diagnoses, NIC interventions, and NOC outcomes within the new common unifying structure.

Since the proposed common unifying structure for NANDA, NIC, and NOC is in the public domain, nurses involved in language development, education, administration and leadership, and clinical practice are encouraged to use the classification. Continued feedback from all nurses will be needed in order to advance nursing language overall and to increase its use throughout the discipline.

References

American Nurses Association. (1995). *Nursing's Social Policy Statement*. American Nurses Publishing.

American Nurses Association. (1998). *Standards of Clinical Nursing Practice, 2nd edition*. American Nurses Publishing.

Dochterman, J. M., & Jones, D. (2001). Collaboration in Nursing Classification: A Conference. National Library of Medicine Conference Grant Proposal, R13 LM07243.

Donaldson, S., & Crowley, D. (1978). The discipline of nursing. *Nursing Outlook, 26*, pp. 113–120.

Gebbie, K., & Lavin, M. (1975). *Proceedings of the First National Conference: Classification of Nursing Diagnoses*. St. Louis, MO: C. V. Mosby Co., p. v.

Jones, D. (1997). Nursing knowledge and outcomes: An integrated perspective. In C. Roy, Sr., & D. Jones (Eds.), *Linking Nursing Knowledge to Practice Outcomes*. Knowledge Conference Proceedings. Chestnut Hill: BC Press, pp. 77–89.

Collaboration in Nursing Classification: The Creation of a Common Unifying Structure for NANDA, NIC, and NOC

2

*NNN August 2001 Conference Group**

For more than twenty-five years, nurses have struggled unsuccessfully to consistently communicate nursing practice to others. The extensive narrative about patient care in the literature includes descriptions about patient behaviors and reactions, along with specific actions taken by nurses to respond to patients' experiences. In recent years, increased attention has been paid to successful outcomes and changes in plans of care. Methods of documentation have varied over the years, with multiple differences observed in terms of both the language and format used to documenting patient care. Streamlined checklists, critical pathways, and problem-oriented charting have been put in place to reduce documentation and respond to changing regulations related to reimbursement.

In the midst of these changes, nurses have created a variety of documentation forms but have been hindered by the lack of a common disciplinary language that effectively communicates patient problems and supporting data, outcomes, and related nursing actions. As a result, nursing practice is poorly communicated to patients/clients, to other nurses, other healthcare providers, and policy makers. The essence of professional nursing lies within the dynamic nurse–patient relationship. It is important that nursing language captures a portion of this experience directly related to patient behaviors and experiences. Nurses worldwide need to be able to use and expand the language they use so that nursing practice can be articulated, evaluated, and included in discussions of cost-effective, quality patient care.

*The members of the NNN conference group whose work is summarized in this chapter are: Joanne McCloskey Dochterman, Dorothy Jones, Sue Moorhead, Kay Avant, Ida Androwich, Gloria Bulechek, Mary Clarke, Martha Craft-Rosenberg, Janice Denehy, Marjorie Gordon, Pauline M. Green, Barbara Head, Marion Johnson, Mary Ann Lavin, Margaret Lunney, Meridean Maas, Anne Perry, Cheryl Reilly, Cindy Scherb, Sheila Sparks, Judith Warren, and Georgia Griffith Whitley.

Funded in part by a grant from the National Library of Medicine (R13 LM07243). Permission to use parts of this chapter should be requested from Joanne Dochterman, University of Iowa College of Nursing, or Dorothy Jones, Boston College.

This chapter presents the process, content, and outcomes of a project funded by the National Library of Medicine (Dochterman & Jones 2001) designed to create a common unifying structure for nursing languages, specifically NANDA, NIC, and NOC. In this chapter, we describe the process used to achieve this goal, and then we present a proposed structure that unifies these languages.

Issues and Challenges in Using Nursing Language Classifications

In 1973, Kristine Gebbie and Mary Ann Lavin held the First National Conference on the Classification of Nursing Diagnoses to present "a clear articulation of those health problems that comprise the domain of nursing and the classification of the problems into a taxonomic system" (Gebbie & Lavin 1975: *v*). Since that time, other classification systems (e.g., Nursing Interventions Classification, Nursing Outcomes Classification) and language data sets (e.g., Nursing Management Minimum Data Set) have been developed to organize and describe nursing diagnoses, interventions, and nursing sensitive patient outcomes and other components of the care episode (e.g., staffing, cost). By 2001, the American Nurses Association had recognized eight nursing classification systems, two nursing data sets, and two nomenclatures (Coenen, McNeil, Bakken, Bickford & Warren 2001).

This proliferation of nursing language classification systems has resulted in a lack of a unified disciplinary language, leading to confusion among nurses in practice across specialties and settings. Although mapping efforts associated with the development and use of terminology models (e.g., SNOMED) are underway, these efforts are designed to relate different languages "behind the computer screens" and are, to date, untested. Even when the reference terminology models are successful for the collection and comparison of nursing data, they do not assist the clinician or student to learn or to use the language at the bedside. The inconsistent use of nursing languages in documenting patient problems and responses has minimized nursing's visibility and compromised the contributions of nurses to quality and cost-effective patient outcomes. Lack of consistent use of nursing language in practice has significantly reduced the integration of nursing language and clinical reasoning approaches into academic curricula across programs. This has led to a growing number of new graduates with limited knowledge of nursing language, culminating in inconsistent documentation of patient problems. Failure to effectively communicate nursing practice has compromised reimbursement and limited nursing's ability to provide policy makers with data needed to change these policies.

In addition, the development of the substantive content for the domain of nursing has been compromised and the growth of the science has been restricted. The problems nurses solve each day when they respond to patients and with multiple populations are poorly articulated. As a result, knowledge development and clinical investigation are negatively impacted. The multiplicity of language classification systems has also decreased the inclusion of nursing language within information systems, further compromising nursing's ability to communicate its disciplinary contributions to patient outcomes. Although nursing has gained the attention of policy makers (Testimony 1999) and there is a willingness to include nursing language in healthcare information systems, system developers also want to harmonize nursing language and move toward a more unified language that is responsive to nurses globally.

Contributions of a Common Unified Structure for Nursing Language

The time has come for development of a common unified structure[1] for nursing language. Within existing terminologies certain points of consensus have been reached, particularly within the North American Nursing Diagnosis Association classification, the Nursing Interventions Classification, and the Nursing Outcomes Classification. Although these three classifications have been linked with each other (Johnson, Bulechek, Dochterman, Maas, & Moorhead 2001), the lack of a common organizing structure does not visually indicate that the three classifications are related. Developers of these structures share common thinking around nursing language and professional nursing. The development of a common unifying structure for these nursing languages will provide significant contributions for nursing knowledge development, clinical practice, education policy, and information systems development. These contributions, which we have culled from the literature and our collective experience, are acknowledged in the following:

For **Knowledge Development** *a unified structure will:*

- Enable scientists to focus on concept development and isolate the essential content of the discipline.
- Contribute to the definition of nursing science and professional nursing practice.
- Support the contributions of language to knowledge development and the development and use of midrange and practice theory.
- Articulate further the phenomena of concern to the discipline and lead to the development of new knowledge.

For **Clinical Practice** *a unified structure will:*

- Improve the articulation of diagnoses, interventions, and outcomes.
- Reduce the complexity of integrating these three elements of nursing care.
- Differentiate more clearly the contributions of the discipline to cost-effective quality care.
- Reflect the complexity of clinical nursing practice.
- Contribute to nursing's visibility in evidence-based practice.
- Help to standardize documentation across settings and improve communication among nurses and other care providers.
- Create movement toward a standardized nursing assessment.

---

[1]The terms *common unified structure, common organizing structure,* and *taxonomic structure* or *taxonomy* have a common meaning in this chapter.

*For **Education** a common unified structure will:*

- Guide faculty in curriculum development and evaluation.
- Foster the integration of language into nursing curricula at all program levels.
- Organize the language of the content of the discipline for teaching clinical decision-making.
- Help to provide graduates with knowledge and expertise for communication of nursing judgments, interventions, and measurement of outcomes.

*For **Research** a common unified structure will:*

- Guide researchers in the development, testing, accuracy, and refinement of nursing diagnoses, interventions, and outcomes.
- Promote the development and testing of predictive models that will link patient outcomes to practice contributions across clinical specialties.
- Facilitate research to identify high-incidence problems that are critical for all nurses to know and resolve.
- Facilitate the integration of nursing knowledge into clinical databases that are used for effectiveness research.

*For **Health Policy** a common unified structure will:*

- Help to integrate nursing information within the electronic patient record and national nursing databases used for health policy decision-making.
- Provide a structured, unified framework for capturing clinical nursing information.
- Help to create an accurate model for administrators and insurers to determine the cost of nursing care.
- Facilitate reimbursement for specific dimensions of nursing practice related to patient problem identification, interventions, and outcomes.
- Help to accurately define provider mix and complexity of patient care used to make patient assignments and assign resources.

*For **Information Systems** a common unified structure will:*

- Create an improved structure for inclusion of nursing language into new and existing information system models.
- Aid in the development of a database that fosters the mapping/linking of diagnoses, interventions, and outcomes across terminology models.
- Improve data access, storage, and retrieval needed by researchers, clinicians, policy makers, and administrators.
- Enable systematic evaluation of existing terminologies and their relevance and use in clinical practice.
- Increase the overall use of nursing languages and long-term viability of NANDA, NIC, and NOC internationally.

The Invitational NNN Conference: Drafting a Common Structure

An invitational conference, funded by a grant from the National Library of Medicine, was held at the Starved Rock Conference Center in Utica, Illinois, August 12–14, 2001. The grant project objectives are listed in Table 2-1. The purpose of the conference was to develop a first draft of a common unified taxonomic structure for the three classifications of the North American Nursing Diagnosis Association (NANDA), the Nursing Interventions Classification (NIC), and the Nursing Outcomes Classification (NOC). Twenty-five participants knowledgeable in the development, testing, and refinement of classification systems were invited to participate in the conference. One participant became ill a few days before the conference and was unable to attend. Representatives from the Omaha and HomeHealth Care systems were among those who were initially invited but later declined the request to participate. The meeting convened with 24 participants, including 22 nurse experts, a keynote speaker, and a staff person (see Chapter Appendix 2.1 for a list of conference participants). The two-day conference agenda is outlined in Table 2-2.

Method Used to Develop a Common Unified Structure

The conference began with a keynote presentation on the science of classification by Geoffrey Bowker, professor in the Department of Communication at the University of San Diego, La Jolla, California. Dr. Bowker has spent his academic career studying the structure of knowledge in various disciplines. His presentation reinforced the need for nursing classifications and placed the current nursing work in the context of the development, articulation, and growth of knowledge. His paper is presented in full in this monograph.

During the first afternoon and morning of the second day, conference participants reviewed the need for a common structure (M. Lunney's presentation is included in this monograph) and the structures of NANDA, NIC, and NOC, as well as other nursing classification systems and data sets currently in use.

TABLE 2-1 Conference Objectives

Language Structure

---

1. Articulate the assumptions underlying each language (diagnoses, interventions, and outcomes).
2. Identify issues that will need to be addressed to achieve a common taxonomic structure.
3. Examine existing taxonomic structures currently in use clinically.
4. Prepare a first draft of a "White Paper" on the common taxonomic structure linking NANDA, NIC, and NOC.
5. Plan strategies for dissemination and feedback of the "White Paper" at venues including an open forum at the April 2002 NANDA, NIC, and NOC conference.

Following dissemination and feedback of the document:

6. Develop a position paper detailing the need for the common structure and the methodology used to develop the proposed structure.
7. Create mechanisms to integrate feedback and to disseminate the final structure to nurses globally.

T A B L E 2 - 2   NNN Conference 2001 Schedule

Sunday, August 12, 2001

Afternoon

1:00	Registration
1:30	*Welcome and Conference Overview* Joanne McCloskey Dochterman and Dorothy Jones
1:45–3:00	*Opening Address: The Science of Classification* Geoffrey Bowker
3:00–3:30	Break
3:30–5:00	*Statement of the Problem*–Joanne McCloskey Dochterman, Moderator Overview of the existing taxonomic structures of NANDA, NIC and NOC Kay Avant, NANDA Gloria Bulechek, NIC Marion Johnson, NOC

Monday, August 13, 2001

Morning

8:00	*Overview of Day* Dorothy Jones
8:30–10:00	*The Need for One Taxonomic Structure: Three Perspectives* Dorothy Jones Margaret Lunney Judy Warren
10:00–10:30	Break
10:30–12:00	*Panel Presentations and Discussion: Overview of Other Relevant Organizing Structures;* *Comparison of these with structures of NANDA, NIC, and NOC; Discussion of Issues* Functional Health Patterns–Marjory Gordon Omaha System–Anne Perry Home Health Care Classification–Barbara Head Others: Patient Care Data Set, Perioperative Data Set, and International Classification of Nursing Practice–Sue Moorhead

Afternoon

12:00–1:00	Lunch
1:30	*Guidelines and Tasks for Smal-Group Work* Joanne McCloskey Dochterman
2:00–5:30	*Small-Group Work*
After Dinner As needed	See Small-Group Instructions

Tuesday, August 14, 2001

Morning

8:30–10:00	*Report of Progress from Groups*
10:00–10:30	Break
10:30–12:00	*Total Group Discussion–Coming to Consensus* Led by Joanne McCloskey Dochterman and Dorothy Jones

Afternoon

12:00–1:00	*Plans for Preparation of Position Paper and Dissemination*
1:00	Conference Adjournment
1:30–4:00	*Post-Conference Meeting–Putting together final draft of one structure* Joanne Dochterman, Dorothy Jones, Kay Avant, Sue Moorhead

Although all participants were familiar with some of the systems, this review helped to assure a common starting place for each conference participant. Discussions relating to each presentation helped to uncover issues and to offer solutions in areas of concern. The time spent examining existing nursing terminologies helped each member establish some common expectations and generated enthusiasm for the current project and the importance of the work at hand.

On the second day, the group was divided into four small work groups, each with an assigned leader and recorder. Before arriving, the participants had received for review the organizing structures of six languages to help create a common structure for NANDA, NIC, and NOC. Participants were also instructed to bring with them to the conference the classification books of NANDA, NIC, and NOC, as well as any other materials, such as a dictionary or thesaurus, that might be helpful in advancing the work of the group.

Overview of the Organizing Structures Reviewed

The six organizing structures on which information was sent to every participant in advance for review were: NANDA's Taxonomy 2, NIC's Taxonomy, NOC's Taxonomy, Gordon's Functional Health Patterns, Home Health Care Classification's 20 components, and the Omaha System's structure. The six structures were selected because they are used frequently in clinical practice. They are commonly acknowledged as "front- end" clinical terminologies useful in helping practicing nurses to plan and document care. Each of the structures selected has an organizing structure thought be helpful to the purpose at hand.

North American Nursing Diagnosis Association (NANDA)—Taxonomy 2

The NANDA Taxonomy 2 (NANDA 2001) was approved for adoption by the NANDA members at their conference in April 2000. It consists of 12 domains (e.g., Health Promotion, Nutrition) and 46 classes (e.g., Health Awareness, Ingestion). Each domain and class has a definition, and a total of 155 diagnoses are included at the third level of the taxonomy.

Nursing Interventions Classification (NIC), 3rd ed.

The NIC taxonomy (McCloskey & Bulechek 2000) consists of 7 domains (e.g., Physiological: Basic, Behavioral) and 30 classes (e.g., Activity and Exercise Management; Coping Assistance). Each domain and class has a definition. The 486 interventions are placed in the classes at the third level of the taxonomy.

Nursing Outcomes Classification (NOC), 2nd ed.

The NOC taxonomy (Johnson, Maas, & Moorhead 2000) consists of 7 domains (e.g., Functional Health, Physiologic Health) and 29 classes (e.g., Energy Maintenance; Growth & Development). Each domain and class has a definition. The 260 outcomes are placed in the classes at the third level of the taxonomy.

Gordon's 11 Functional Health Patterns

The Functional Health Patterns (Gordon 1994) contain 11 pattern areas (e.g., nutrition-metabolic, health perception–health management, elimination) and are used by numerous educators, students, and clinicians to organize the nursing assessment data and information from physical examination to arrive at nursing diagnoses. Gordon has organized the NANDA diagnoses into 11 patterns, and the new NANDA Taxonomy 2 domains reflect a modification of the Functional Health Patterns.

Home Health Care Classification (HHCC)

The 145 diagnoses and 160 interventions in this system (Saba, 1992) were developed for home healthcare nurses to use in practice and are classified in 20 categories (e.g., Activity, Bowel Elimination, Cardiac, Cognitive). The classification reflects diagnoses, interventions, and outcomes. The 20 components are at the class level of some of the other classifications and may be helpful in the design of a common structure.

Omaha System

The Omaha System, developed in the mid-1970s for use in community health (Martin & Scheet 1992), contains three schemes for problems, interventions, and outcomes. Forty problems are organized in four domains: environmental, psychosocial, physiological, and health-related behaviors. The intervention scheme consists of four broad categories (e.g., the first category is health teaching, guidance, and counseling) and 62 targets for intervention. The outcome ratings are measured by using three 5-point scales for the concepts of knowledge, behavior, and status.

Small-Group Work: Guidelines for a Common Structure

The small-group work began following a review and discussion of nursing languages and presentations from group members. There was a general session in which one of the group leaders presented guidelines for constructing a common structure. This information had been prepared in advance of the conference and was based on personal experience and the literature. Table 2-3 presents the "Guidelines for Constructing a Common Organizing Structure: The Desiderata" for consideration and use by groups as they deliberated on developing a common unified structure for nursing language. (The word "desiderata" and some of the content were adopted from the article by Cimino [1998].)

In the small-group sessions that followed this presentation, each group (Table 2-4) was asked to work through the development of a draft of a common structure according to written instructions found in Table 2-5. Participants were told that they could deviate from the instructions if they thought another approach would achieve the outcome, that is, a draft of a common structure.

Each group worked independently throughout the afternoon and into the evening. Individuals demonstrated a readiness for the task at hand and a willingness to take the next step: the creation of a common taxonomic structure. Although differences of opinion arose, these differences were addressed through discussion, compromise, and consensus. The next morning each group presented its unique picture of a common unified structure, with a clear rationale for the perspective taken.

T A B L E   2 - 3   **Guidelines for Constructing a Common Organizing Structure: The Desiderata**

The users of the proposed structure will include:

1. Developers of NANDA, NIC, and NOC and other nursing classifications.

2. Practicing nurses, students, and other clinicians who wish to locate a particular diagnosis, intervention, or outcome.

3. Developers of information systems who will use the structure to organize screens.

4. A host of others, including faculty, for use in courses and curriculum design, researchers, and policy makers.

Ten Desiderata for Developers:

1. *Simplicity of Structure:* Keep the structure simple—two levels above the concept label level seems to work, naming them domains and classes.

2. *Parsimony of Groups:* The second level (classes) should be around 25 to 30 groups; first level (domains) under 10. More than this is hard to handle mentally and is beyond what can be easily put on a computer screen.

3. *Clear Language:* The names of the groups (domains and classes) should be clear, short (three words or fewer), and descriptive enough to know what kinds of diagnoses, interventions, and outcomes are included.

4. *Formal Definitions:* Each domain and class should have a definition.

5. *Distinct Groups:* The structure should minimize need/desire to cross-reference; classes/domains should be distinct so that diagnoses, interventions, and outcomes can preferably be placed in only one location.

6. *Graceful Evolution:* The structure should resonate with users; be similar to what is now familiar so that the move to new structure is relatively easy.

7. *Domain Completeness:* An "other" category (not elsewhere classified) should *not* be included.

8. *Theory Neutral:* The structure should be useful in any institute, nursing specialty, or care delivery model regardless of philosophical orientation.

9. *Other Discipline Friendly:* Headings (domains and particularly classes) should preferably be recognizable and useful for all disciplines—e.g., process and body system.

10. *Scientific Common Sense:* The structure should look and feel scientific but also reflect common sense.

T A B L E   2 - 4   **Work Group Member Assignments**

Group A	Group B
Martha Craft-Rosenberg, Leader	Gloria Bulechek, Leader
Pauline M. Green, Recorder	Sheila Sparks, Recorder
Mary Clarke	Kay Avant
Dotty Jones	Marion Johnson
Meridean Maas	Cheryl Reilly
Judy Warren	

Group C	Group D
Cindy Scherb, Leader	Georgia Whitley, Leader
Mary Ann Lavin, Recorder	Janice Denehy, Recorder
Ida Androwich	Joanne Dochterman
Marjorie Gordon	Anne Perry
Barbara Head	Sue Moorhead
Margaret Lunney	

TABLE 2·5 Directions for Group Work

Instructions: You are encouraged to plan your time carefully so that you address
the languages and have adequate time to complete number 4.

Select two of the organizing structures (NANDA, NIC, NOC, Functional Health Patterns, Home Health Care, Omaha) and:

Step 1. 30 minutes

Identify a few assumptions underlying the structures you are working with and identify considerations that need to be addressed using these as the basis for a common structure.

Step 2. 30 minutes

Review the selected taxonomic structures and try to fit some examples from the NANDA, NIC, and NOC languages. (For example, if you have chosen NANDA, try to fit NIC and NOC; if you have Gordon, fit examples from NANDA, NIC, or NOC.)

Step 3. 30 minutes

Identify any issues and problems that arise. What modifications can be made to make the structure work, or should another approach be taken?

Step 4. 90 minutes

Propose a draft of a common taxonomic structure, including some examples. This draft can be a modification of an existing structure or a totally new structure. Include examples of placement of NANDA diagnoses, NIC interventions, and NOC outcomes.

Assumptions: Two of the four work groups spent part of their time identifying the assumptions on which a combined taxonomic structure for NANDA, NIC, and NOC would be based. One of the groups identified four assumptions, whereas the other group identified nine assumptions. The following list combines the ideas of both groups.

1. Nursing classifications (NANDA, NIC, and NOC) describe the phenomena of nursing practice and represent the clinical judgments nurses need to make.
2. Nursing classifications represent the knowledge base of nursing and relate to all settings and specialties.
3. Nursing classifications are useful for clinical practice, education, research, and administration.
4. The nursing classifications are advanced enough to identify key concepts that can be harmonized.
5. The classifications need to address individual, family, community, and health system dimensions.
6. Classifications evolve and change as nursing changes, and a structure can evolve to handle these changes.
7. Classifications can capture the holistic nature of nursing's perspective.

Issues: Several issues were obvious at the beginning of the discussion in the work groups. The two principal ones were:

1. Dealing with their own sense of "territoriality" regarding the various languages represented. Participants had to agree upfront in the dialogue that each person would keep an open mind and would try to think in terms

of what the best overarching structure would be, regardless of personal or professional inclinations. This proved to be surprisingly easy once the small-group work began. The various language developers were pretty evenly divided in each group, allowing everyone to have a say in the product of the group but with no language predominating.

2. Concern about composing a framework that encompassed "patient-focused concepts" with "nurse-focused concepts." Some of the participants voiced a concern that it was not appropriate to combine patient-focused diagnoses and outcomes with nurse-focused interventions. Others felt that since all three (diagnoses, interventions, and outcomes) are in the domain of nursing, an overarching framework could encompass all three. After some discussion, they agreed that if they didn't try, they would never know. By the time all the groups had completed their work, there was a general consensus that a unifying structure was possible and that, although the approaches by each group were different, the final initial drafts of structures had many similarities.

Results: One group produced a list of new classes for all three structures, another group identified new classes and domains, while a third group placed the current classes of NANDA, NIC, and NOC in a modified version of the Gordon Functional Health Pattern structure. A fourth group identified new domains and placed the current classes in these domains according to type of recipient (i.e., individual, family, and community). Each of these drafts was discussed in terms of the issues and challenges it presented.

The final session of the third day was spent identifying the common challenges and the direction the group desired to take on each challenge. For example, the group was unanimous in its desire that the new structure include both new classes and new domains in which the labels of all three classifications could be placed. Although the importance of family and community was acknowledged, the majority of participants did not want to see these as domains. There was total agreement that the terms used should clearly communicate the type of concepts included and that the words used should be familiar to clinicians. On the third day of the conference, the group adjourned in high spirits at mid-day, expressing their feelings that they had accomplished a lot and that they believed that, though a perfect document was not possible, a final draft of one common structure could be achieved.

Post-Conference Activity: Synthesizing a Common Structure

Immediately following the conference, a small-work group [Joanne Dochterman (NIC), Dorothy Jones (NANDA), Sue Moorhead (NOC), and Kay Avant (NANDA)] met for the afternoon to prepare a first draft of the proposed structure based upon the work of the four groups and the general discussion for the two days. Owing to the structure of NANDA, it was desirable to have both the current president of NANDA (Kay Avant) and the past president and co-organizer of this conference (Dorothy Jones) participate in the post-conference activities.

Following a brief discussion of the four proposed structures from the conference work groups, the post-conference task force decided that a first step would be to compare the two drafts of new classes with each other as well as with the modified Gordon classes prepared by a third group. When this was done, a number of similarities were noted—although named differently, the same classes were identified. The task force discussed each of the alternative names and selected the one that communicated the best or chose a new name. The end result of this exercise was 28 potential classes.

The next step was to organize these classes into domains. One group at the conference had produced four new domains that were well received by the participants. The task force used these four domains plus one other suggested in the discussion as the initial starting point for the domains of the common structure. Each of the 28 classes was then placed in the five domains. At this point the five domains were labeled Health/Life Style, Physiological Function, Psychosocial Function, Life Principles, and Environment/Health Protection.

As the process evolved, some of the classes were thought to be relevant to two of the domains, with the greatest amount of redundancy seen between Health/Life Style and Physiological Function as well as Health/Life Style and Psychosocial Function. For example, the classes of Activity/Exercise and Sleep/Rest were initially placed in both Health/Life Style and Physiological Function. After discussion of these and other classes placed in two locations, each class was placed in only one location, where it was thought to fit best. The placement was helped by the definitions of each domain which the post-conference group generated. As work progressed, it became apparent that the proposed domain of Life Principles was overlapping with the domain of Health/Life Style, and since the Life Principles domain had only one class in it (Values/Beliefs, which includes spirituality), it was decided to combine these domains calling them, at this time, Health/Life Styles.

After some editing, a new proposed structure consisting of four domains (Health/ Lifestyle, Physiological, Psychosocial, and Environment/Health Protection) and 27 classes was created. The task force reviewed each of the issues that were raised by the four conference groups against the proposed structure and determined that the proposed structure had addressed each of the concerns. For example, various participants strongly indicated that the new structure must be able to accommodate "growth and development," medications, and the care in the community.

A few months after the conference, this draft of the proposed unified common structure was sent to each conference participant for review and feedback, along with a set of questions that addressed particular aspects of the proposed structure (e.g., Should the Comfort class be divided into two classes—Physical Comfort and Physiological Comfort—and then be placed in different domains?) Based on the participants' comments, changes were made in the proposed structure. For example, the word "health" was taken out of the titles of two of the domains and two of the classes, with the rationale that all of this pertained to health. Definitions of two of the domains and some of the classes were changed, and titles of some classes were changed. All changes were made in the interest of keeping the practicing nurse in mind and focusing on what the practitioner would find most helpful and easiest to understand.

The 2002 NNN Conference: Presenting the Proposed Structure

At the April 2002 NNN conference in Chicago, the structure was disseminated and there was further discussion by a larger community. During this conference, attended by over 300 individuals from the United States and nearly a dozen other countries, a plenary session was held, with 90 minutes devoted to presentation of the process used, the proposed structure, and discussion. All participants had copies of the draft of the paper and proposed structure, and a lively discussion ensued. One suggestion was to post the paper and structure on the web and to allow more time for feedback. One week after the conference, the paper and structure were posted on the web sites of both NANDA and the Center for Nursing Classification and Clinical Effectiveness, and the feedback was requested via the Center's listserv. Based on the feedback presented during the discussion period at the conference and the responses received from the web postings, the paper and structure were again revised. Among the major changes were a change in the name of the first domain from lifestyle to functional; a change in the definitions of three of the domains and several of the classes; the addition of the emotional class; and a name change from safety promotion class to risk management. Several other minor changes were made to reduce wordiness and to improve consistency in format. (Chapter Appendix 2.2 contains a summary of the comments on drafts 2 and 3 and the resulting changes that were made in each round. Chapter Appendix 2.3 acknowledges the individuals and groups that gave verbal or written feedback on draft 3.)

Although several of the issues raised have been resolved by the changes in names and definitions, some differences of opinions remain that cannot be reconciled in one structure; the revised structure will not be entirely to everyone's liking. This is the nature of consensus. It is also the nature of nursing—nurses work in a variety of settings with different philosophical orientations and levels of skill. The effort to achieve a common structure to account for all of nursing practice is a tall order. Nonetheless, we believe that the result is a very good beginning—a harmonization of all views has been accomplished.

Proposed Taxonomy of Nursing Practice

The proposed structure, consisting of 4 domains and 28 classes, integrates the work of all participants and work groups at the conference and takes into account the reflection and feedback of the participants following the conference (see Table 2-6). This structure is different from the existing structures of NANDA, NIC, and NOC, and yet is not a radical departure from any of them. This is considered desirable inasmuch as it favors none and at the same time forms an effective transition to the use of a common structure. The structure is also in the public domain, available for use by any group or individual.

The proposed structure meets the desired guidelines (see Table 2-3) for a common structure. The two-level structure is simple, consistent with existing structures, and will be easy for clinicians to use. The number of classes

TABLE 2-6 Taxonomy of Nursing Practice

Domains			
I. Functional Domain Includes diagnoses, outcomes, and interventions to promote basic needs.	**II. Physiological Domain** Includes diagnoses, outcomes, and interventions to promote optimal biophysical health.	**III. Psychosocial Domain** Includes diagnoses, outcomes, and interventions to promote optimal mental and emotional health and social functioning.	**IV. Environmental Domain** Includes diagnoses, outcomes, and interventions to promote and protect the environmental health and safety of individuals, systems, and communities.

Classes			
includes diagnoses, class outcomes, and interventions that pertain to:			
Activity/Exercise—Physical activity, including energy conservation and expenditure.	**Cardiac Function**—Cardiac mechanisms used to maintain tissue profusion.	**Behavior**—Actions that promote, maintain, or restore health.	**Health Care System**— Social, political, and economic structures and processes for the delivery of healthcare services.
Comfort—A sense of emotional, physical, and spiritual well-being and relative freedom from distress.	**Elimination**—Processes related to secretion and excretion of body wastes.	**Communication**—Receiving, interpreting, and expressing spoken, written, and nonverbal messages.	**Populations**—Aggregates of individuals, or communities having characteristics in common.
Growth and Development— Physical, emotional, and social growth and development milestones.	**Fluid and Electrolyte**— Regulation of fluid/electrolytes and acid base balance.	**Coping**—Adjusting or adapting to stressful events.	**Risk Management**—Avoidance or control of identifiable health threats.
Nutrition—Processes related to taking in, assimilating, and using nutrients.	**Neurocognition**—Mechanisms related to the nervous system and neurocognitive functioning, including memory, thinking, and judgment.	**Emotional**—A mental state or feeling that may influence perceptions of the world.	
Self-Care—Ability to accomplish basic and instrumental activities of daily living.	**Pharmacological Function**— Effects (therapeutic and adverse) of medications or drugs and other pharmacologically active products.	**Knowledge**—Understanding and skill in applying information to promote, maintain, and restore health.	
Sexuality—Maintenance or modification of sexual identity and patterns.	**Physical Regulation**—Body temperature, endocrine, and immune system responses to regulate cellular processes.	**Roles/Relationships**— Maintenance and/or modification of expected social behaviors and emotional connectedness with others.	
Sleep/Rest—The quantity and quality of sleep, rest, and relaxation patterns.	**Reproduction**—Processes related to human procreation and birth.	**Self-Perception**—Awareness of one's body and personal identity.	
Values/Beliefs—Ideas, goals, perceptions, spiritual, and other beliefs that influence choices or decisions.	**Respiratory Function**— Ventilation adequate to maintain arterial blood gases within normal limits.		
	Sensation/Perception—Intake and interpretation of information through the senses, including seeing, hearing, touching, tasting, and smelling.		
	Tissue Integrity—Skin and mucous membrane protection to support secretion, excretion, and healing.		

This structure is in the public domain and can be freely used without permission; neither the structure nor a modification can be copyrighted by any person, group, or organization; any use of the structure should acknowledge the source.

The papers in the monograph are copyrighted by the authors, and permission to use parts of the papers should be sent to the authors.

(parsimony of groups) is not overwhelming. The names for domains and classes are clear, and each has a formal definition. The names will also be familiar to members of other disciplines, thereby allowing for use across disciplines if desired. All classes are listed in only one domain. The classification is theory neutral and may be used with any philosophical orientation as well as any specialty or care delivery model.

The structure was developed so that the NANDA, NIC, and NOC developers (as well as others, if desired) could place their diagnoses, interventions, and outcomes in these same classes and domains. Initially, these are likely to be separate publications (each using the same structure), but over time, and perhaps with some modifications, the three languages can be placed together and published together in the one structure.[2] Information systems can use the one structure to help students and practicing nurses to locate and select the appropriate diagnosis, intervention, or outcome. The use of one common structure should facilitate the identification of linkages between diagnoses, interventions, and outcomes and thus encourage research that examines the relationships. Nursing curricula can be designed using the structure as a framework. It is also possible that, in time, the structure's 28 classes will evolve into a common assessment tool usable by all nurses to collect and communicate patient data.

Conclusion

Having a nursing language facilitates communication between nurses and with the providers. Using nursing language can promote:

- Describing the substantive content of the discipline,
- Defining the in elements of care and assigned a cost based upon parameters such as complexity and acuity,
- Developing a database that can be analyzed and used to predict staffing mix and care requirements, and
- Articulating the focus of nursing practice and nursing's unique contributions to patient care outcomes to other disciplines.

When nursing care is documented with standardized language, the resulting data can be aggregated and studied. The results of nursing care are known.

Changes in practice can be made based on the results of research that was real clinical data. New avenues of research using clinical databases based on the documentation, actual care delivered and outcomes achieved are opened. Nurses can study the cost and effectiveness of care.

The proposed "Taxonomy of Nursing Practice" (Table 2-6) is a structure specifically designed for the integration of NANDA, NIC, and NOC, but it can also be used by other language developers and others who desire to organize

---

[2]At the time we submitted this manuscript for publication, it was our understanding that the developers of NANDA, NIC, and NOC had each agreed that they would place their diagnosis, intervention, or outcome concepts in their forthcoming editions of the classifications.

or index nursing content. Within this proposed framework, gaps in language about the human experience and the nurse patient/client relationship can be identified and studied. The presentation of diagnoses, interventions, and outcomes in one unifying structure will facilitate the teaching and use of the languages and further the goals of the profession as they relate to delivering and assuring quality patient care. We believe that this effort in collaboration and harmonization is one more step toward a preferred future.

References

Cimino, J. J. (1998). Desiderata for controlled medical vocabularies in the twenty-first century. *Methods of Information in Medicine, 37*, 394–403.

Coenen, A., McNeil, B., Bakken, S., Bickford, C., & Warren, J. J. (2001). Toward comparable nursing data: American Nurses Association criteria for data sets, classification systems, and nomenclatures. *Computers in Nursing, 19* (6), 240–246.

Dochterman, J. M., & Jones, D. (2001). Collaboration in Nursing Classification: A Conference. National Library of Medicine Conference Grant Proposal, R13 LM07243.

Gebbie, K., & Lavin, M. (1975). *Proceedings of the First National Conference: Classification of Nursing Diagnoses.* St. Louis, MO: C V. Mosby Co., p. v.

Gordon, M. (1994). *Nursing diagnosis: Process and application.* New York: McGraw-Hill.

Gordon, M., Avant, K., Heardman, H., et al (Eds.) (1999). *Nursing diagnoses: Definitions and classification 2001–2002.* Philadelphia: North American Nursing Diagnosis Association.

Johnson, M., Bulechek, G., Dochterman, J. M., Maas, M., & Moorhead, S. (2001). *Nursing diagnoses, outcomes, interventions: NANDA, NOC, and NIC linkages.* St. Louis, MO: Mosby Year Book.

Johnson, M., Maas, M., & Moorhead, S. (Eds.) (2000). *Nursing Outcomes Classification (NOC).* 2nd ed. St. Louis, MO: Mosby Year Book.

Martin, K. S., & Scheet, N. J. (1992). *The Omaha System: Application for community health nursing.* Philadelphia: Saunders.

McCloskey, J. C., & Bulechek, G. M. (Eds.) (2000). *Nursing Interventions Classification (NIC).* 3rd ed. St. Louis, MO: Mosby Year Book.

North American Nursing Diagnosis Association (NANDA). (2001). *Nursing diagnoses: Definitions and classification 2000–2001.* Philadelphia: NANDA.

Saba, V. K. (1992). The classification of home health care nursing: Diagnoses and interventions. *Caring Magazine, 11* (3), 50–57.

Testimony presented at the National Committee on Health and Vital Statistics-Sub Committee (NCVHS). (1999).

NNN 2001
Conference Participants

The conference participants included:

1. *Ida Androwich,* PhD, RN, FAAN, Professor of Nursing and Director of Informatics, Center for Nursing Research, Niehoff School of Nursing, Loyola University in Chicago, IL. Dr. Androwich has a clinical background in ambulatory and home health care nursing. She was the Site Co-ordinator for Loyola for the NIC implementation study from 1993–1996 and has conducted two studies on the use of NIC interventions in ambulatory care. She is also on the Steering Committee for the National Nursing Vocabulary Summit.

2. *Kay Avant,* PhD, RN, FAAN, Associate Professor, University of Texas–Austin, TX. Dr. Avant is the current President of the North American Nursing Diagnosis Association. Her work has focused on language development and nursing diagnosis. She has served as the Chairperson of the NANDA Taxonomy Committee and has helped craft the newly approved Taxonomy II. Her publications relate to theory and concept development. She has knowledge about the standards and structure of nursing language and experience in the development and use of conceptual frameworks in nursing.

3. *Geoff Bowker*, PhD, Professor in the Department of Communication at the University of San Diego, La Jolla, CA. He has spent his academic career studying the structure of knowledge in various disciplines. He presented the keynote talk of the conference on the science of classification and assisted in laying important groundwork for collaboration.

4. *Gloria Bulechek*, PhD, RN, FAAN, Professor at the University of Iowa College of Nursing. She is co-principal investigator (with McCloskey Dochterman) of the Nursing Interventions Classification (NIC). She has a background as a clinical specialist in the acute care setting and as a teacher of advance practice nurses. She has many years of expertise in language development and research methodology.

5. *Mary Clarke*, MA, RNC, Informatics Nurse Specialist, Genesis Medical Center in Davenport, IA, is familiar with issues related to the implementation in practice and information systems of all three languages. Her facility is one of the premier clinical institutions in the country to have implemented NANDA, NIC, and NOC in a clinical nursing information system. Mary is a member of NANDA, and is a member of both the NIC and NOC research teams.

6. *Martha Craft-Rosenberg*, PhD, RN, FAAN, Professor at the University of Iowa College of Nursing, is a member of the Nursing Interventions Classification research team and the co-chair of the NDEC (Nursing Diagnosis Extension Classification) research team that has a collaborative contract with NANDA to refine and develop nursing diagnoses. She is serving in her second term on the NANDA taxonomy committee. She has a clinical background in Pediatrics and contributes expertise in family nursing and language development.

7. *Janice Denehy*, PhD, RN, Associate Professor at the University of Iowa College of Nursing, is a member of the Nursing Interventions Classification research team and the co-chair with Martha Craft-Rosenberg of the NDEC (Nursing Diagnosis Extension Classification) research team that has a collaborative contract with NANDA to refine and develop nursing diagnoses. She has a background in family nursing and is editor of the national journal on School Nursing.

8. *Joanne McCloskey Dochterman*, PhD, RN, FAAN, Distinguished Professor and Director of the Center for Nursing at the University of Iowa College of Nursing, is co–Principal Investigator (with Gloria Bulechek) of the Nursing Interventions Classification (NIC). She is a past member of the NANDA Board of Directors and co-chair of the NNN Alliance. She has also participated in the national efforts to develop a Reference Terminology Model for nursing. She has an extensive research and funding background in the areas of nursing administration and classification. She has participated in various efforts to link NIC and NOC with NANDA.

9. *Marjorie Gordon*, PhD, RN, FAAN, Professor Emerita, Boston College, Boston, MA, was the first President of NANDA and is currently a member of the Board of Directors. She has served as Co-Chair of the NANDA Diagnostic Review Committee and has helped to establish standards for reviewing new submissions for inclusion in the NANDA Taxonomy. Dr. Gordon has written and presented numerous workshops on clinical judgment. She is the author of a seminal textbook on nursing diagnosis that organizes the diagnoses by a conceptual framework known as functional health patterns.

10. *Pauline Green*, PhD, RN, is Associate Professor at Howard University in Washington, DC. She has a background in adult health nursing and intensive care nursing. She has been active in NANDA and has multiple publications on a variety of topics, including environmental nursing diagnoses and the diagnosis of high risk for injury.

11. *Barbara Head,* PhD, RN, Assistant Professor, University of Nebraska Medical Center, Omaha, NE. For 3 years Barb served as Research Associate, Center for Nursing Classification at the University of Iowa College of Nursing, responsible for running the day-to-day activities of the Center and assisting with the upkeep of NIC and NOC. She has a strong practice background in community health nursing and has participated in research efforts to link NIC and NOC to NANDA.

12. *Marion Johnson,* PhD, RN, Professor Emerita at the University of Iowa College of Nursing, is the co–Principal Investigator (with Maas and Moorhead) of the Nursing Outcomes Classification (NOC). She has participated in national efforts to develop a Reference Terminology Model in nursing and in efforts to link NOC with NANDA and NIC. She has a background as a clinical specialist and long experience and interest in outcomes measurement. She has an extensive publication and funding record in quality of care and classification research.

13. *Dorothy A. Jones,* EdD, RNC, Professor, Boston College, Boston, MA, is the immediate Past President of NANDA; she serves as Co-Chair of the NNN Alliance. She brings her work in knowledge development, nursing informatics and language development to this project. Dr. Jones has conducted multiple funded research projects that helped to identify nursing phenomena (interventions and outcomes) within a variety of clinical populations. In addition, she has developed and established the psychometric properties of the Functional Health Pattern Assessment Screening Tool (FHPAST), which uses as a conceptual framework the work of Gordon (1994). Dr. Jones has authored numerous publications in the area of nursing language.

14. *Mary Ann Lavin,* DSc, RN, FAAN, Associate Professor, Saint Louis University, St. Louis, MO, is president-elect of NANDA and currently a Board member of the Association. She s the co-founder of the NANDA Nursing Diagnosis Association. She brings a long history with nursing language development and diagnosis research, particularly with primary care populations. Dr. Lavin is a nurse practitioner and developer of a project called LINKS, which allows nurses from around the world to dialogue about nursing languages, particularly nursing diagnosis. She is a growing expert in the area of informatics and nursing language.

15. *Margaret Lunney,* PhD, RN, Professor and Program Coordinator, Master of Science in Adult Health Nursing at the College of Staten Island, City University of New York, has a long involvement in NANDA and numerous publications on nursing diagnosis and critical thinking. Dr. Lunney completed an NIH funded study of the effects of using NANDA, NIC, and NOC on the health outcomes of school children. Her clinical and teaching background is in adult health and community health.

16. *Meridean Maas*, PhD, RN, FAAN, Professor at the University of Iowa College of Nursing, is the co–Principal Investigator (with Johnson and Moorhead) of the Nursing Outcomes Classification (NOC). She has an impressive research and publication background in gerontology, long-term care administration, and language development. She was on the NIC research team during the early stages of development and is currently on the NANDA Board and serves as Secretary of the Association.

17. *Sue Moorhead*, PhD, RN, Associate Professor at the University of Iowa College of Nursing, is co–Principal Investigator (with Johnson and Maas) of the Nursing Outcomes Classification (NOC). Dr. Moorhead is also a member of the NIC research team and a member of NANDA. She has been involved in various efforts to link NANDA, NIC, and NOC. She teaches informatics and nursing administration courses at Iowa.

18. *Anne Perry*, EdD, RN, FAAN, Professor, St. Louis University, St. Louis, MO, is a new member of the NANDA Board of Directors. She has long been affiliated with the work of language development, implementing nursing diagnosis in clinical practice and teaching students the relevance, utilization and evaluation of nursing diagnosis within the academic setting. She is the co-author of a widely used nursing fundamentals book, now in its fifth edition.

19. *Cheryl Reilly*, PhD, RN, is a Corporate Manager in the Clinical Systems Research and Development Group at Partners HealthCare System in Chestnut Hill, MA. She is leading the development of an automated patient assessment application that aims to capture structured information for facilitating decision support and quality monitoring. Her research in informatics has focused on taxonomy development, assessing the ability of standardized vocabularies to represent nursing concepts in a computer-based patient record, care planning systems, and capturing patients' assessments of their signs and symptoms.

20. *Cindy Scherb*, PhD, RN, is Patient Care Documentation and Informatics/Research Coordinator at Immanuel St. Joseph's–Mayo Health System in Mankato, MN. At this site she has led the implementation of NANDA, NIC, and NOC in a computerized patient record. She is working on her doctoral dissertation, which is the conduction of effectiveness research using a database with standardized language. She is familiar with each of the languages and the needs of clinical practice.

21. *Sheila Sparks*, DNSc, RN, FAAN, Director and Associate Professor, Shenandoah University Division of Nursing, Winchester, VA, currently serves as Treasurer of NANDA and is a member of its Board of Directors. Dr. Sparks has long been affiliated with the work of language development and nursing diagnosis. She is the author of a major textbook, *Nursing Diagnosis Reference Manual* (2000), currently in its 5th edition, and has conducted research in the area of rehabilitation nursing, with special emphasis on skin care and patient outcomes for persons with spinal cord injuries.

22. *Judith Warren*, PhD, RN, FAAN, Associate Professor, University of Nebraska School of Nursing, has been a long time scholar in the area of nursing diagnosis and language development overall. She is active with groups such as Health Level 7 and has been assigned by the American Nurses Association to be their representative to SNOMED. Dr. Warren's role is to assist in the development of a reference terminology for SNOMED across nursing languages. She has been involved with the international community on developing standards for computerizing nursing language within information systems.

23. *Georgia Griffith Whitley*, EdD, RN, Professor Emerita, Northern Illinois University, DeKalb, IL, is a long time regional, national and international member of nursing diagnosis groups. She currently serves on the NANDA Board of Directors and is the Board liaison to the Research and Diagnosis Review Committee. Dr. Whitley has received funding at the national level for research in language development and has been a facilitator of nursing diagnosis in both clinical and academic settings. She has skill in concept development, research methodologies and language development. Dr. Whitley is currently employed as a group therapist at the National Behavioral Center in Joliet, Illinois.

24. *Ken Cleveland*, BS, CSEd, is the Account Executive with Resource Management Plus (Nursecom), the company that is responsible for the business operations of NANDA. He provided staff assistance at the conference.

Comments on Drafts 2 and 3 and Resulting Changes

Comments on Draft 2

Paper was sent only to conference participants.

Responses to Questions Posed:

Can the Sexuality class be omitted and combined with the Self-Perception class?
Almost everyone said no; no change.

Should the Comfort class be divided into 2 classes: Physical Comfort, put in the Physiological Domain, and Emotional Well-Being, put in the Psychosocial Domain?
About half said yes and half said no—those that said no felt pretty strongly; no change for now.

Is the class Health Behaviors repetitive/overlapping of other classes and, thus, could be omitted?
People wanted this class separate, but the title with Health in it was troublesome (why health here and not other places?); retitled Behavior Change and moved to Psychosocial Domain.

Should the class Life Cycle Processes be called Growth and Development to make it clearer?
Nearly everyone said yes; change made.

Can any of the classes in the Health/Lifestyle Domain be moved to the Psychosocial Domain?
Many said no, some said yes and made specific suggestions. This domain was retitled Lifestyle Domain with a definition change, and 2 classes then moved to Psychosocial.

Summary of Major Changes:

Titles of Domains I and IV were changed—Health wording taken out. (One participant made a strong case that it is all health and to have two domains with this title in it was a bias—she also wanted Health taken out of two of the class names, which was done.)

Domain I and III definitions were changed—Domain I is the more "normal," and the other domains are more those that are trying to get back to normal or optimal; the word emotional was changed to mental in Domain 3 definition as suggested by a couple of individuals.

Health Behavior and Health Knowledge classes changed to Behavior Change and Knowledge and moved to Psychosocial Domain—Makes for a more even distribution of classes and, with definition changes of domains, fits better here.

Cognitive class was changed to Neurocognitive with a refinement of definition— To ensure that neurological has a place and to make this more physiological (but the class physical functioning may need to be changed now).

Definitions of several classes were changed/modified/improved—Suggestions that made changes that used definitions by certain authors or that were excessively wordy were not used. A few suggestions that would require a whole new reconception of this were also not used. All changes were made trying to keep the practitioner user in mind and what they would find most helpful/easiest to understand. All in all, reviewers liked the new structure. There were differences of opinions on some things; some of everyone's suggestions were used.

Comments on Draft 3

The paper was distributed to the 300+ participants at the NNN conference in April 2002 and posted on two web sites for the following two months.

Summary of Major Comments and Changes Made:

Name of Lifestyle Domain is troublesome—Implies choice and choice is not always part of what is included here; also represents a very "Western" view; Please look at International Classification of Function, Disability, and Health (ICF) especially at the top domain level—function is a preferred term

    Change: Domain name changed to Functional and definition changed.

Same comfort issue again—Some want split; some do not.

    No change

Definitions of some classes troublesome—Cardiac Function, Fluid and Electrolyte Pharmacological Balance, Physical Regulation, Coping.

    Change: Definitions of these classes were changed.

Question as whether to combine or not to combine the Cardiac and Respiratory classes

    No Change: Left as separate as there are too many concepts (diagnoses, interventions, and outcomes) to fit in just one class.

Neuro appears in two places: Neurocognitive and Physical Regulation.

    Change: Taken out of Physical Regulation.

Suggestion that the class Nutrition should be moved to the Physiological Domain.

No Change: Class not moved but definition changed to make this be more basic.

Population class—A bit different type of group—Doesn't fit under Environmental Domain. Is the Environment Domain about safety? Others want population class kept. Overlap between Safety and Population.

Change: Definition of Environment Domain changed to include safety and class of Safety Protection changed to Risk Management.

Where is Emotion??

Change: A new class, Emotional, was added.

Individuals and Groups Who Gave Comments on Draft 3

Several individuals gave feedback on the paper, either verbally during the conference forum or in writing during the following months.

We acknowledge the following people for their feedback:

Laurie Baker	Mary Killeen
Suzanne Beyea	Scott Lamont
Rosemary Carroll-Johnson	Mary Ann Lavin
Susan Chase	Marge Lunney
Tania Chianca	Carrol Lutz
Martha Craft-Rosenberg	Karen Martin
Jeanette Daly	Geri Meyer
Pauline Green	Sue Moorhead
Marcy Harris	Nico Oud
Crystal Heath	Kathy Parrish
Lois Hoskins	Gunn von Krogh
Marion Johnson	Bonnie Wakefield
Jane Kelley	Judy Warren

American Nurses Association Committee for Nursing Practice Information Infrastructure (Victoria Elfrink, Suzannne Beyea, Linda Goodwin, Gail Keenan, Barbara McNeil, Judy Ozbolt, Susan Pierce, Linda Thede)

Theoretical Explanations for Combining NANDA, NIC, and NOC

3

Margaret Lunney

The nursing classifications systems of NANDA, NIC, and NOC are language systems designed to represent three interacting and cyclical elements of nursing care: diagnoses, interventions, and outcomes. The relevance and applicability of each of these systems are enhanced with use of the other two systems. Because the three languages were developed by three different groups, their hierarchical structures of domains and classes differ from one another. Differences in the structures of the three systems make it difficult for users to identify the interrelationships among the three systems. Efforts to develop a common structure for these three systems have practical utility, but theoretical explanations for a new structure are also needed because the usefulness of standardized nursing languages (SNLs) to quality-based nursing care has been challenged (Hagey & McDonough 1984; Leininger 1990; Mitchell 1991; Shamansky & Yanni 1983; Smithbattle & Diekemper 2000, 2001) and the time and effort to initiate these systems should be justified. This chapter explains why theoretical explanations for using SNLs are needed and describes the relevance of three theoretical perspectives: linguistics theory, critical thinking, and accuracy of nurses' diagnoses to discern interventions and outcomes.

Need for Theoretical Explanations

Two of the explanations currently used to support use of SNLs are that they are needed to document diagnoses, interventions, and outcomes in the electronic health record and to increase the visibility of nursing's contributions to healthcare events. These explanations are inadequate to sell the idea of NANDA, NIC, and NOC because they are viewed as self-serving for nursing. Nurses and others who reject the idea of standardization, as well as the complexity and cost of implementation, need theoretical explanations for use of standardized nursing languages.

Even though there are many nurse supporters of SNLs such as NANDA, NIC, and NOC, there are also many nurses who criticize their use. The lack of support can be damaging and may prevent widespread adoption of SNLs. One harmful response is covert; that is, nurse leaders and members of other disciplines in healthcare agencies, education, and research ignore and avoid SNLs. These responses may be based on reluctance to learn what is considered a "fad," lack of funds to buy books and software for learning and teaching about these systems, lack of acceptance that an electronic health record will be mandated, belief that SNLs do not fit with selected theories and research, and assumptions that standardization of terms causes harm to patients and does not represent holistic nursing care.

A few negative responses occasionally surface in nursing journals, which reinforce the negative views of SNLs (Hagey & McDonough 1984; Leininger 1990; Mitchell 1991; Shamansky & Yanni 1983; Smithbattle & Diekemper 2000, 2001). In addition, nurses on computer-based listservs periodically discuss the advantages and disadvantages of SNLs. Nurses who support SNLs generally point out that nursing care needs to be visible in the healthcare system rather than explaining the relevance to quality-based nursing care, while nonsupporters claim that the quality of nursing care is better without standardized nursing languages.

As a result of these objections and criticisms, SNLs are not included in agency-based information systems, not used for documentation of diagnoses, outcomes, and interventions, not included in nursing curricula, and not studied by nurse researchers. Combining NANDA, NIC, and NOC will address some, but not all, of the objections or criticisms of standardized nursing languages. Supporters of NANDA, NIC, and NOC can use theory to explain why development and use of SNLs are essential for the progress and growth of the discipline and how use of SNLs contributes to quality-based nursing care.

Theoretical Explanations for NNN

Three theoretical perspectives show the importance of using standardized nursing languages to achieve positive healthcare outcomes. These are Hayakawa's *linguistics theory* (Hayakawa & Hayakawa 1990), *critical thinking perspectives* (Brookfield 1991; Scheffer & Rubenfeld 2000), and the *concept of accuracy of nurses' diagnoses* (Lunney 2001).

Linguistics Theory

Linguistics theory proposes that languages such as the scientific classifications of NNN are fundamental mechanisms of survival and the most highly developed of symbolic processes (Hayakawa & Hayakawa 1990). Scientific classifications are necessary tools for communication with self and others. Nurses, like other people, think with words, so they need words to think about the phenomena of concern. Nurses may not even discern events for which they have no words or phrases to think.

Communication with self and others enables nurses to combine the strengths and abilities of their neurological systems with that of others, increasing the energy and talents that are available for decision-making and problem solving. According to Hayakawa and Hayakawa (1990), scientific classifications are tools to improve human experiences. The availability of classification systems enables nurses to work collaboratively with individuals, families, and communities, other nurses, and members of other disciplines. By standardizing the meanings of terms, people can speak more clearly with one another as they work on healthcare issues of concern.

Scientific names are needed because word usage varies by region (Hayakawa & Hayakawa 1990). Even from one unit to another unit in a hospital setting, nurses may be using different terms for the same meanings and the same terms for different meanings. Naming is considered a great step forward because it makes discussion possible.

Linguistics theory tells us that there are no "right" names for anything (Hayakawa & Hayakawa 1990). Yet, some of the stated objections to use of nursing diagnoses relate specifically to the words or phrases that are used; for example, the names are too obtuse (Shamansky & Yanni 1983), do not reflect the nature of nursing (Mitchell 1991), or do not reflect the culture of the patient (Leininger 1990). Linguistics theory reminds us that the existing names of classification systems should be used until better names are proposed and accepted. The names of classification systems evolve over time to meet the needs of the group—that is, the nurses and the consumers whom they serve.

According to linguistics theory, naming is classifying so that every time a name is given to a phenomenon, classification is occurring. This means that, even without standardization of terms, classification occurs. The advantage of standardizing the names of a nursing classification is that nurses can communicate more clearly with healthcare consumers and one another. Standardization enables the sharing of information to explain phenomena. The criticism that nursing diagnoses do not portray the health "process" (Mitchell 1991) is not relevant because naming anything at any time, no matter what the name is, captures only static parts of any process. Hayakawa and Hayakawa (1990) explain the process of a living cow and its complexity, showing that we cannot even capture the essence of a cow with the words we use. Humans automatically abstract from their experiences to identify the similarities among events, not the differences. Figure 3-1 illustrates the various levels of abstractions as they

FIGURE 3-1 Abstraction Ladder (Read from bottom up)

8. Healthy Society

7. Child welfare

6. Parenting

5. Decision-Making Processes

4. Nursing Diagnosis: Decisional Conflict re: Infant Feeding Choice

3. Partnership process

2. Cheryl's' observed breastfeeding behaviors

1. Experience of breastfeeding

Possible Abstractions for a Nursing Case Study on Breastfeeding (Gigliotti & Lunney, 1998).

relate to a nursing event described by Gigliotti and Lunney (1998). Nurses, like other humans, continually abstract from experiences in order to think about them, so it makes no sense to distrust abstractions (Hayakawa & Hayakawa 1990).

Classifications are developed for specific purposes. For a science such as nursing, classifications represent pooled knowledge and further contribute to the pooling of knowledge (Hayakawa & Hayakawa 1990). The research processes used to develop this pooled knowledge are described in the NIC and NOC books (Johnson, Maas, & Moorhead 2000; McCloskey & Bulechek 2000), and for the NANDA nursing diagnoses (North American Nursing Diagnosis Association 2001) in a wide variety of sources, such as the *International Journal of Nursing Language and Classification* and conference proceedings books.

Pooled nursing knowledge helps nurses to deal with the physical world of nursing. As a complex scientific field, the more knowledge that is available for nurses, the more likely that nurses will be able to find ways to help consumers. Smithbattle and Diekemper (2000, 2001) expressed concern that use of taxonomies and protocols is antithethical to experience in the complex world of nursing. If this were so, it would be an incorrect use of standardized languages. Classifications accomplish their goals only when they are used in conjunction with clinical experiences. The meanings of words are known through context, and context is gained only through experience. Words must always be connected to the events for which they stand. Any nurse who uses SNLs needs to be sure that he or she avoids words describing words and instead connects the words of these classification systems to the real world of nursing. Use of case studies for teaching SNLs is one way to keep the words of NANDA, NIC, and NOC connected to the physical world of nursing.

Connecting standardized languages to the physical world of nursing is important because words always have extensional and intensional meanings (Hayakawa & Hayakawa 1990). Extensional relates to the meanings that exist in the physical world—that is, the meanings of consumers, other nurses, and members of other disciplines. Intensional relates to individual connotations. Individual connotations of every word and phrase are used in relation to healthcare events. An advantage of using the words and phrases of SNLs is that nurses' inferences and decisions are exposed to the scrutiny of others. In contrast, prejudice occurs if nurses focus only on their own connotations and do not share their thoughts with others. The words and phrases of NNN should be used in partnership with healthcare consumers so that the terms that "best fit" the clinical situations are selected for use.

The words and phrases of nursing classification systems are maps to the territory of nursing (Hayakawa & Hayakawa 1990). Many maps are needed to know a territory, and no map fully represents the territory. All maps together do not equal the territory. Mitchell (1991) proposed that the NANDA diagnoses do not adequately represent the nature of nursing phenomena, and Hayakawa and Hayakawa (1990) would certainly agree. No processes, even those that are much less complex than nursing events, can be adequately represented with words and phrases. It is impossible, then, for any words to fully represent any phenomenon.

FIGURE 3-2 Language and Power in the Nursing Process

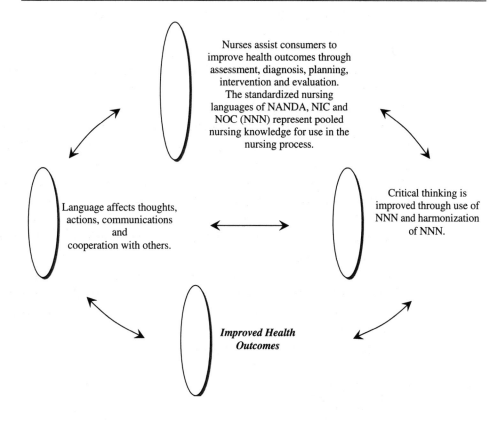

Nurses assist consumers to improve health outcomes through assessment, diagnosis, planning, intervention and evaluation. The standardized nursing languages of NANDA, NIC and NOC (NNN) represent pooled nursing knowledge for use in the nursing process.

Language affects thoughts, actions, communications and cooperation with others.

Critical thinking is improved through use of NNN and harmonization of NNN.

Improved Health Outcomes

Science seeks generally useful classifications that produce results. Results in nursing should be quality-based nursing services. The quality of nursing care will be improved through use of SNLs such as NANDA, NIC, and NOC because the availability of pooled nursing knowledge and opportunities for increased communication and cooperation will improve nurses' thinking, which, in turn, will improve nurses' actions on behalf of patients (Figure 3-2).

The goal of classification is to make good maps of the territory of nursing. For NNN, harmonization is the next step in making good maps. Combining NNN will make it easier to use these systems, which, in turn, will increase nurses' experiences of connecting these words and phrases to the real world of nursing. Combining these systems makes it easier to depict the interrelationships among diagnoses, interventions, and outcomes, and reduces the complexity of identifying interventions and outcomes that relate to specific diagnoses.

Critical Thinking Perspectives

Critical thinking perspectives can also be used to explain the importance of using NANDA, NIC, and NOC and the harmonization of these three systems. Brookfield (1991) described critical thinking as an important part of being a developing person. Brookfield's four components and five phases of critical thinking can be enhanced through use of standardized nursing languages. The four components are (pp. 7–9):

1. Identifying and challenging assumptions is central to critical thinking.
2. Challenging the importance of context is crucial to critical thinking.
3. Critical thinkers try to imagine and explore alternatives.
4. Imagining and exploring alternatives leads to reflective skepticism.

Use of the concepts in NANDA, NIC, and NOC helps nurses to challenge assumptions, imagine alternatives, and use reflective skepticism because these systems are much more comprehensive (i.e., there are almost 900 concepts in the three systems) than anything nurses can consider without them. Research has substantiated that human beings can only consider 7 ± 2 bits of data in short-term memory (Newell & Simon 1972) so, without access to comprehensive lists of standard terms, nurses mentally generate short lists of possible diagnoses, interventions, and outcomes from memory. When used correctly, these systems are used in the context of experience and with consideration of the contexts of clinical situations. Thus, use of these systems may also enhance nurses' abilities to challenge the importance of context.

According to Brookfield (1991), the five phases of critical thinking are (pp. 26–29):

1. A trigger event prompts discomfort and perplexity.
2. Appraisal of the event leads to identification of a concern and perusal of possibilities.
3. Exploration of the mind and other resources generates new ways of examining discrepancies and testing answers, concepts, and so forth.
4. Development of alternative explanations helps the person to make sense of the situation.
5. New ways of thinking and acting are integrated into the fabric of the person's life.

The cues in clinical situations trigger nurses' awareness of a need to decide what is the consumer's problem, risk state, or readiness for health promotion. In phase two, identification of a concern is likely to be more accurate with the availability of a large number of concepts. In phase three, examination of the mind and other resources will be more efficient and effective with harmonization of NANDA, NIC, and NOC. Harmonization makes it easier to find and use the related concepts of diagnoses, interventions, and outcomes. In phases four and five, the nurse has many more options to consider with use of the almost 900 concepts in NANDA, NIC, and NOC, as well as consideration of concepts that are not included in NANDA, NIC, and NOC. One of the concerns with use of standardized languages is that nurses will only use concepts within the system and may "force fit" patient situations into existing but inadequate concepts. This would be an incorrect use of these systems. Concepts that are not in these systems should be used as indicated and, if found to be useful, should be submitted to developers of these systems for possible inclusion in one of these systems.

The dimensions of critical thinking in nursing were identified through a Delphi study of 57 nurse experts (Scheffer & Rubenfeld 2000; Table 3-1). A majority of the cognitive skills and habits of mind identified through this study

TABLE 3-1 Critical Thinking in Nursing: Definitions of Terms*

Dimensions of Critical Thinking	Definitions
Cognitive Skills	
Analyzing	Separating or breaking a whole into parts to discover the nature, function and relationships.
Applying Standards	Judging according to established personal, professional, or social rules or criteria.
Discriminating	Recognizing differences and similarities among things or situations and distinguishing carefully as to category or rank.
Information Seeking	Searching for evidence, facts, or knowledge by identifying relevant sources and gathering objective, subjective, historical, and current data from those sources.
Logical Reasoning	Drawing inferences or conclusions that are supported in or justified by evidence.
Predicting	Envisioning a plan and its consequences.
Transforming Knowledge	Changing or converting the condition, nature, form, or function of concepts among contexts.
Habits of the Mind	
Confidence	Assurance of one's reasoning abilities.
Contextual perspective	Consideration of the whole situation, including relationships, background, and environment, relevant to some happening.
Creativity	Intellectual inventiveness used to generate, discover, or restructure ideas; imagining alternatives.
Flexibility	Capacity to adapt, accommodate, modify, or change thoughts, ideas and behaviors.
Inquisitiveness	An eagerness to know by seeking knowledge and understanding through observation and thoughtful questioning in order to explore possibilities and alternatives.
Intellectual integrity	Seeking the truth through sincere, honest processes, even if the results are contrary to one's assumptions and beliefs.
Intuition	Insightful sense of knowing without conscious use of reason.
Open-mindedness	A viewpoint characterized by being receptive to divergent views and sensitive to one's biases.
Perseverance	Pursuit of a course with determination to overcome obstacles.
Reflection	Contemplation upon a subject, especially one's assumptions and thinking for purposes of deeper understanding and self-evaluation.

*Scheffer, B. K., & Rubenfeld, M. G. (2000). A consensus statement on critical thinking. *Journal of Nursing Education, 39,* 352–359.

can be improved through exposure to the pooled knowledge represented in NANDA, NIC, and NOC. Improvement of critical thinking processes will improve the outcomes of thinking, that is, decisions about the elements of nursing care and the actions taken by nurses in response to these decisions.

Six of the seven types of cognitive skill processes may be more efficient and effective with use of the terms from NANDA, NIC, and NOC and with harmonization of the three systems.

1. *Analyzing* the relationships of *patient cues* to inferences/diagnoses and of diagnoses to interventions and outcomes is easier with the availability of these research-based lists of diagnoses, interventions, and outcomes.
2. *Analyzing* the relationships of *diagnoses* to outcomes and interventions will be more efficient when NNN is organized in a common structure.
3. *Discriminating* the meaning of data is supported by the availability of definitions and descriptions with these systems.

4. The processes of *information seeking* as it pertains to diagnoses, outcomes, interventions, and interrelationships are stimulated by the availability of pooled knowledge in NNN.

5. *Applying standards* for quality-based holistic care is facilitated through the identified connections between diagnoses, interventions, and outcomes.

6. Nurses' use of *logical reasoning* for decision-making is more efficient when diagnostic, intervention, and outcome concepts are organized in systematic ways.

7. The processes of *predicting* plans of care and quality-based outcomes of care are broader and more comprehensive with the availability of pooled knowledge in NNN.

Nurses, like all other human beings, think with words, so thinking is facilitated through the availability of words that describe nursing phenomena. The standardization of definitions and descriptions of the meanings of these concepts facilitates communication of thinking processes with others and connection to the thinking of others. Collaboration with others in critical thinking helps nurses to achieve accurate diagnoses of human responses and discernment of the best interventions and outcomes.

Accuracy of Nurses' Diagnoses

An outcome of critical thinking is accuracy of interpreting the cues in clinical situations in order to identify client problems, risk states, or readiness for health promotion. Accuracy of nursing diagnosis is a "rater's judgment of the degree to which a diagnostic statement matches the cues in a client situation" (Lunney 1990). Accuracy in nursing was described as a continuous variable, not a dichotomous one. This is because the phenomena that nurses diagnose are overlapping and are not discretely different from one another. For example, powerlessness is closely related to ineffective coping, problems with tissue integrity are closely related to poor nutritional status, and ineffective breathing pattern is closely related to impaired gas exchange. Thus, some diagnoses may be close to high accuracy, while other diagnoses may be judged as low accuracy. A seven-point scale from high to low accuracy can be used to measure the accuracy of nurses' diagnoses (Lunney 2001). The characteristics of accuracy of nurses' diagnoses are listed in Table 3-2.

Accuracy is particularly important because diagnostic choices guide the selection of interventions and outcomes, whether or not nurses formally use diagnostic concepts from NANDA and other systems. With human limitations regarding short-term memory, nurses continually must infer the meaning of data. Some of these inferences are diagnoses, whether or not they are named as such. Nurses who do not formally use diagnostic languages such as NANDA have an even greater risk of being inaccurate than nurses who use these languages. With formal use of a diagnostic language, nurses have more opportu-

TABLE 3-2   Characteristics of Accuracy of Nurses' Diagnoses*

▮ Accuracy of a nursing diagnosis is relative to the interactive elements in a client situation.

▮ The challenge of achieving high levels of accuracy ranges from simple to complex depending on the numbers of cues, types of cues, and characteristics of cues.

▮ Accuracy includes the use of supporting and conflicting cues.

▮ High degrees of accuracy of nursing diagnoses are the result of integrating all the obtainable cues to make as precise a statement as possible.

▮ The stringency of achieving accuracy is relative to the situation.

▮ Low-accuracy diagnoses reflect one or more of the following characteristics:
    Use of unreliable or invalid cues
    Ignorance or misinterpretation of conflicting cues
    Lack of integration of relevant cues for other diagnoses
    Evidence that another diagnosis is more likely
    Lack of agreement with the client or other experts on the phenomenon in question.

*Lunney, M. (1990). Accuracy of nursing diagnosis: Concept development. *Nursing Diagnosis, 1*, 12–17.

nities to reflect on diagnostic choices, and other persons have opportunities to confirm or challenge diagnostic choices.

In a review of research findings pertaining to the accuracy of nurses' diagnoses (Lunney 2001), it was exquisitely clear that low-accuracy interpretations may regularly occur. For example, in a study in which nurses agreed to have the accuracy of their diagnoses judged by two clinical experts (Lunney, Karlik, Kiss, & Murphy 1998, reprinted in Lunney 2001), only 45.2% of the psychosocial diagnoses of 153 newly admitted patients by 62 staff nurses in three hospitals were judged as the two highest levels of accuracy. On the seven-point scale of accuracy, almost 13% of diagnoses of the 153 cases were judged as the three lowest levels of accuracy. In this study, nurses' accuracy was probably higher than usual because they knew they were being judged for accuracy. Low levels of accuracy occur because of the complexity of diagnosing human responses and are probably exacerbated by a lack of attention to accuracy in clinical agencies, nursing education, and nursing research (Lunney 1999, reprinted in Lunney 2001).

Because low accuracy diagnoses logically lead to inappropriate choices of interventions and outcomes, any factor that has potential to improve nurses' accuracy (e.g., use of standardized nursing languages and harmonization of NANDA, NIC and NOC) should be implemented to improve health outcomes.

Discernment of the most appropriate interventions and outcomes is also challenging for nurses considering the complexity of human beings and the comprehensive responsibilities of nurses to help people with health promotion, health protection, and health restoration. Clinical situations differ widely, based on many contextual factors—for example, culture, age, and medical history. The contextual factors that relate to clinical situations affect critical thinking processes and need to be considered when deciding what are the best interventions and outcomes. With so many contextual factors and so many possible interventions and outcomes to consider, discernment of the most appropriate categories will be facilitated by the harmonization of NANDA, NIC, and NOC.

Summary

Linguistics theory explains that naming a scientific phenomenon is important for "knowing" about that phenomenon. The standardized names in NNN are maps to the territory of nursing. These maps are not perfect, but linguistics theory tells us that there are no right names for anything. Supporters of NNN can mitigate criticisms by clarifying that the labels of NNN are *not* nursing—rather, they are only abstractions based on the similarities among events, not the differences—and by explaining the connections of NNN to thinking and actions. Nurses should use the available names in NNN until better ones are created and available for use.

The reality of naming is that names do not fully reflect a phenomenon, even the simplest of events. Yet, names are essential for thinking and subsequent actions. Use of the standardized terms from NNN facilitates improvements in nursing care by fostering collaboration and cooperation among nurses, consumers, and other providers. It is important to connect the names of NNN to the physical world of nursing through case studies.

Critical thinking processes and outcomes are improved with use of NNN and harmonization of NNN. Accuracy of nurses' diagnoses are important because selection of the most appropriate interventions and outcomes are based on the nurses' inferences from client data.

Nurses can explain the importance of using NNN and the relevance of combining NNN into one structure through use of linguistics theory, critical thinking perspectives, and the outcomes of critical thinking. These theoretical perspectives can be used to show the relationship of using NNN to quality-based nursing care and as a basis for research studies. Research is needed to provide empirical support for these theoretical perspectives.

References

Brookfield, S. D. (1991). *Developing critical thinkers: Challenging adults to explore alternative ways of thinking and acting.* San Francisco: Jossey-Bass.

Gigliotti, E., & Lunney, M. (1998). Integration of Neuman's Systems Model with the theory of nursing diagnosis in postpartum nursing. *Nursing Diagnosis, 9* (14), 34–38.

Hagey, R. S., & McDonough, P. (1984). The problem of professional labeling. *Nursing Outlook, 32*, 151–157.

Hayakawa, S. I., & Hayakawa, A. R. (1990). *Language in thought and action* (5ᵗʰ ed). San Diego, CA: Harvest Original, Harcourt & Brace.

Johnson, M., Maas, M., & Moorhead, S. (Eds.). (2000). *Nursing Outcomes Classification (NOC), Iowa Outcomes Project* (2ⁿᵈ ed.). St. Louis, MO: Mosby.

Leininger, M. (1990). Issues, questions, and concerns related to the nursing diagnosis cultural movement from transcultural nursing perspective. *Journal of Transcultural Nursing, 2*, 23–32.

Lunney, M. (1990). Accuracy of nursing diagnosis: Concept development. *Nursing Diagnosis, 1*, 12–17.

Lunney, M. (2001). *Critical thinking and nursing diagnosis: Case studies and analyses.* Philadelphia: North American Nursing Diagnosis Association.

McCloskey, J. C., & Bulechek, G. M. (Eds.) (2000*). Nursing Interventions Classification (NIC), Iowa Interventions Project* (3rd ed.). St. Louis, MO: Mosby.

Mitchell, G. J. (1991). Diagnosis: Clarifying or obscuring the nature of nursing. *Nursing Science Quarterly, 4* (2), 52.

Newell, A., & Simon, H. (1972). *Human problem solving.* Englewood Cliffs, NJ: Prentice-Hall.

North American Nursing Diagnosis Association. (2001). *Nursing diagnoses: Definitions and classification, 2001–2002.* Philadelphia: Author.

Scheffer, B. K., & Rubenfeld, M. G. (2000). A consensus statement on critical thinking. *Journal of Nursing Education, 39,* 352–359.

Shamansky, S. L., & Yanni, C. R. (1983). In opposition to nursing diagnosis: A minority opinion. *Image, 15* (2), 47–50.

Smithbattle, L. & Diekemper, M. (2000). A wrong turn: How taxonomies lead nursing astray. *American Journal of Nursing, 100* (7), 9.

Smithbattle, L., & Diekemper, M. (2001). Promoting clinical practice knowledge in an age of taxonomies and protocols. *Public Health Nursing, 18,* 401–408.

The Science and Art of Classification | 4

Geoffrey C. Bowker

Introduction

Information work is key to conducting any large enterprise today—it constitutes most of the work for most of us in the United States, whatever line of business we are in (Castells 1996). Information work provides multiple bridges between worlds, such as between the environmental scientist and the policy maker. Thus, we might need to know how many species there are in a given ecosystem in order to make a decision about what land to designate a park. Central to this information work is the ability to classify—to put items into categories so that they can be managed effectively.

The example just given evokes several different classification systems. What is a species? The more precision you ask for (and you need precision in order to build information systems), the less certainty you get. Any of the intuitive species definitions we might use—ability to reproduce sexually with and only with other members of the species; sharing a common genetic heritage; and so forth—is open to question. Some philosophers today argue that the concept of *species* (let alone genus, family, or kingdom) is fundamentally flawed. However, you cannot just get away with a definition of species. You also need to define an ecosystem—and depending on your scientific persuasion, you will give very different definitions—and not only its conceptual definition but its geographic boundaries. Finally, even entities like *parks* can be very hard to define: you need to know whether you are dealing with a world heritage site or a national, state, city, or community park: each come bundled with its own sets of standards and regulations. A central tension for many classification systems in the world of networked information is that they serve multiple purposes. The same species list can be used by scientists to study an ecosystem and by policy makers to determine which species to declare endangered. A given classification of ecosystems might be shared between evolutionary theorists, paleontologists, and population biologists (each with somewhat different constituencies). Although different groups of scientists can agree on the broad delineations of a classification system (e.g., the Linnaean binomial system for plants and animals), they rarely agree on the details. The science of classification is the process of drawing on specialty knowledge in a given area in order to determine the best possible representational apparatus for an activity. The art of classification is the ability to produce an apparatus that can work for the multiple uses for which it will be deployed. Over the past 10 years since its emergence, the NIC classification system has impressed observers both by the science and the art of its architects. They have developed rigorous methodologies for garnering the most detailed picture of the field of nursing possible. In doing so, they have practiced the careful art of drawing in the widest possible community base—making the system work for as many as possible.

In this chapter, the example of the Nursing Interventions Classification (NIC) is presented in order to show the work that was done in developing the system, and then conclusions are drawn about the art of classification.

The Nursing Interventions Classification (NIC) Overcomes Erasure of Nursing Work

The NIC system had two main goals: (1) to help build a knowledge base for the development of scientific nursing and for teaching; and (2) by documenting and representing nursing work in the form of atomic, indivisible units, to promote both the integration of nursing informatics into medical informatics and the recognition of heretofore invisible nursing work by hospital information systems, accounting information systems, and the electronic medical record (Berg & Bowker 1997). Only work that is visible in the information system can truly be identified as valuable—and exact a charge! (Thus, a hospital bill typically records every action of the doctors individually, with nursing work often lumped into the price of the room).

On the other hand, visibility has inherent dangers. Many nurses feel that the classification cannot properly reflect the process-oriented nature of their work. Furthermore, such a representation risks exposing nursing to process re-engineering that could result in the reassignment of the "unskilled" portions of nursing work. The NIC team (see LaDuke 2000, for a concise, readily accessible overview of the NIC and for practice-based examples of its use) has developed a rich strategy for dealing with the central tension between the desire for—and the dangers of—visibility. Managing the tension between visibility and discretion has necessitated that the definition of nursing intervention must itself map the shifting boundaries among direct, indirect, and administrative care, depending on ever-changing concerns surrounding the need for increased legitimacy against the fear of undermining surveillance. Moreover, to protect local autonomy and legitimize local differences, NIC architects have decided to specify only down to the level of interventions, leaving the subactivities of care activities indeterminate and opaque. As Bowker and Star (1999) state: "Common practice, contingency, and legitimacy temper visibility" (p. 248).

This chapter should be considered complementary to other work in nursing classification, such as McCormick and Jones (1998). In their paper, the authors discuss the implications of new technologies for linking classifications at local, network, and universal levels. Particularly relevant to the tone of the present work is their use of the Rosetta Stone as an evocative, resonant metaphor for evolving classifications and nomenclatures.

Nursing work has traditionally been invisible, and its traces have been expunged at the earliest opportunity from the medical record. Nurses themselves have accomplished this externally, by hospital administrations, and internally.

External Erasure

Historically, the selective erasure of nursing records within hospital information systems has been drastic. Nursing records are the first destroyed when a patient is released. The hospital administration does not require them (in accounting, the cost of nursing is frequently lumped in with the price of the room); doctors consider them irrelevant to medical research; and nursing theorists are not well enough entrenched to demand their collection. Nursing has been seen as an intermediary profession that does not need to leave a trace—in accord with traditional gender expectations, nurses are "on call" (Star & Strauss 1999).

Huffman (1990: 319), in a standard textbook on medical records management, writes:

> As nurses' notes are primarily a means of communication between the physicians and nurses, they have served their most important function during the episode of care. Therefore, to reduce the bulk and make medical records less cumbersome to handle, some hospitals remove the nurses' notes from records of adult patients when medical record personnel assemble and check the medical record after discharge of the patient. The nurses' notes are then filed in chronological order in some place less accessible than the current files until the statute of limitations has expired, and they are destroyed.

Traditionally, nurses have been facilitated out of the equation: though they may not have an official trace of their own past, their duty is to remember for others. In one of those vague but useful generalizations that characterize information statistics, a book on next-generation nursing information systems asserted that 24 percent of total hospital operating costs were devoted to information handling. Nursing, it is stated, "accounted for most of the information handling costs (28 percent to 34 percent of nurses' time)"; what is worse, "in recent years, external regulatory factors, plus increasing organizational and health care complexity, have augmented the central position of information in the health care environment" (Zielstorff et al. 1993: 5).

The nursing profession acts as a distributed memory system for doctors and hospital administrators. Nurses manage much of the institutional memory (keeping charts updated, filling forms) and much of the local memory (who needs such-and-such an item and where you can get hold of it). Ironically, in so doing, they have in the past been denied their official memory.

Internal Erasure

Even when the erasure has not been mandated, it has been voluntary. As a motif of the profession, one text on a nursing classification system cites the following observation: "'The subject of record-keeping has probably never been discussed at a convention without some agitated nurse arising to ask if she is expected to neglect her patients in order to write down information about them'" (Martin & Scheet 1992: 21, echoing a 1917 source). And Joanne McCloskey Dochterman, one of the two principal architects of NIC, notes that "the most convincing argument against nursing service or Kardex care plans is the absence of them. Although written care plans are a requirement by the Joint Commission for Hospital Accreditation and a condition for participation in Medicare, few plans are, in fact, written" (McCloskey 1981: 120).

In her study of the International Classification of Diseases, Ann Fagot-Largeault (1989) notes the same reluctance on the part of doctors to spend time accurately filling in a death certificate (itself a central tool for epidemiologists) when they might be helping live patients. Because accurately representing the activities that compose nurses' work takes time, systems are designed to favor summary (e.g., forms) over complex, but more faithful, representations. In the case of a computerized NIC, the NIC implementation team sometimes suspects nurses of using the choices that appear before them on a screen (which they can elect with a light pen) rather than searching through the system for the apt descriptor (from notes taken at Iowa Intervention Project meeting, June 8, 1995).

One of the nurses' main problems lies in their efforts to situate their activity visibly within an informational world that has factored them out of the equation. Furthermore, it has been maintained that they should be so excluded, since what nurses do can be defined precisely as that which is not measurable, finite, packaged, or accountable. In nursing theorist Jenkins's terms: "Nurses have functioned in the post–World War II era as the humanistic counterbalance to an increasingly technology-driven medical profession" (Jenkins 1988: 92). Nursing informaticians face a formidable task. They have tried to define nursing as something that fits naturally into a world partly defined by the erasure of nursing and other modes of invisible articulation work.

Sometimes for these reasons, the nurses are driven by their own logic to impeach medical truth. At other times, they challenge orthodoxy in organization science, or they seek to restructure nursing so that these challenges will not be necessary. At the end of the day, there will be an information infrastructure for medical work that contains an account of nursing activity. Enabled by new information technologies, the move to constant monitoring of work practice (integrated into accounting systems and management information systems) is overwhelming in this profession as in many others. With projects like NIC, which offer new classification systems to embed in databases, tools, and reports, we get to see what is at stake in making invisible work visible.

The Importance of Classification

The very establishment of NIC necessitated that the slate be wiped clean; that is, it required clearance. Prior to its establishment, there was, for example, no standard (i.e., universally accepted) terminology to record nursing interventions. One nursing informatician ruefully noted:

> It is recognized that in nursing, overshadowed as it is by the rubrics of medicine and religion, no nurse since Nightingale has had the recognized authority to establish nomenclature or procedure by fiat. There are no universally accepted theories in nursing on which to base diagnoses, and, in fact, independent nursing functions have not yet gained universal acceptance by nurses or by members of other health professions. (Castles 1981: 40)

Nursing, it was argued, had until then been a profession without form. There was no way of codifying past knowledge and linking it to current practice. A conference was held to establish a standardized nursing minimum data set (information about nursing practice that would be collected from every care facility). The conference found that: "The lists of interventions for any one condition are long partially because nursing has a brief history as a profession in the choosing of interventions and lacks information for decision-making. As a profession, nursing has failed to set priorities among interventions; nurses are taught and believe they should do everything possible" (McCloskey & Bulechek, 1992: 79).

In the face of the view that the nurse does everything that nobody else does, should all previous nursing knowledge be abandoned? William Cody, in an open letter sent to the Iowa Intervention Team that produced NIC and published in *Nursing Outlook* in 1995, charged that this was precisely what would follow from widespread adoption of NIC:

> It would appear that the nursing theorists, who gave nursing its first academic leg to stand on, as it were, are deliberately being frozen out. I would like to ask Drs. McCloskey and Bulechek, Why is there no substantive discussion of nursing theory in your article? How can you advocate standardizing "the language of nursing" by adopting the language of only one paradigm? (Cody, 1995: 93)

The Project team responded that indeed the stakes were high:

> The Iowa group contends that taxonomic development represents a radical shift in theory construction in which the grand conceptual models are not debated, but transcended. We believe that, as a scientific community, nursing has moved to the point of abandoning the conceptual models of nursing theorists as forming the science base of the discipline (McCloskey, Bulechek, & Tripp-Reimer 1995: 95).

Cody's letter and the response underline the importance of the classification work being done. A new language, a new form of communication, was being developed for nurses, and the stakes are always high when you define a language.

It is not just at the level of nursing theory that this act of classification was seen as unsettling. Practicing nurses implementing NIC at one of four testbed sites had several complaints. They stated that learning to use NIC, together with the new computer system of which it was a part, was like going to a foreign country where you had to speak the language; to make matters worse, you had to go to a new country every day. More prosaically, some said that they felt they were going from being experts to novices. The art of classification involves not only negotiating the language but also motivating others to learn it. There is a hope that with the classification scheme nothing vital will be lost in the future and that this goal is worthy of the journey. In the case of NIC it surely is worthy.

Conclusion: The Art of the Science of Classification

The development of a new information infrastructure for nursing, at least part of which the NIC represents, will make nursing more memorable. If the infrastructure is designed so that nursing information must be present as an independent, well-defined category, then nursing itself as a profession will have a better chance of surviving through rounds of business process reengineering, and nursing science as a discipline will have a firm foundation. The fate of nursing, as both profession and discipline, is inextricably intertwined with that of infrastructure projects like NIC: "Having ensured that all nursing acts are potentially remembered by any medical organization, the NIC team will have gone a long way to ensuring the future of nursing" (Bowker & Star, 1999: 275).

A key feature of the ongoing integration of information systems into vast federated systems—be these in government, industry, or the medical professions—is that work which is not represented in those systems is at a huge disadvantage: it cannot be evaluated, accounted for, and/or rewarded. The kind of accounting that goes on frequently involves quantification; in John King's phrase, in general nowadays "numbers beats no numbers every time, even if the numbers one produces are inherently problematic" (personal communication; see also Kraemer, Dickhoven, et al. [1987], for the supporting arguments.) You need to produce numbers (even if you don't fully subscribe to the numbers that you are producing).

The NIC team has displayed great subtlety in developing their scientific classification of nursing work. In both discussions and publications, they have recognized that nursing work is not easily quantifiable and divisible; they have also developed a classification system that retains a judicious level of ambiguity—they do not try to overspecify the parts of a particular intervention. The attempt to produce a scientific classification of nursing work represents one important direction for building up robust nursing knowledge. At the same time, it also represents a significant strategy for defending the profession of nursing. Nursing is in this way no different from any other profession. Andrew Abbott (1988) demonstrates how many modern professions (drawing on the medical model) seek to carve out for themselves an autonomous territory of scientific knowledge. The resulting visibility of nursing work is a boon; the price of that visibility is as yet uncertain.

The classifications of nursing diagnoses, interventions, and outcomes are vital to the future development of the nursing profession and to the development of robust nursing knowledge. Key to the successful completion of this work is skill at both the science and the art of classification.

References

Abbott, A. (1988). *The system of professions: An essay on the division of expert labor.* Chicago: University of Chicago Press.

Berg, M., & Bowker, G. C. (1997). The multiple bodies of the medical record—towards a sociology of the artifact. *The Sociological Quarterly, 38* (Summer 1), 513–537.

Bowker, G. C., & Star, S. L. (1999). *Sorting things out: Classification and its consequences.* Cambridge, MA: MIT Press.

Castells, M. (1996). *The rise of the network society.* Cambridge, MA: Blackwell Publishers.

Castles, M. R. (1981). Nursing diagnosis: Standardization of nomenclature. In H. H. Werley and M. R. Grier (Eds.), *Nursing information systems.* New York: Springer, p. 36–44.

Cody, W. K. (1995). Letter from William K. Cody. In *Nursing Outlook, 43* (2), 93–94.

Fagot-Largeault, A. (1989). *Causes de la mort : Histoire Naturelle et Facteurs de Risque.* Paris : Librairie Philosophique J. Vrin.

Huffman, E. (1990). *Medical record management.* Berwyn, IL: Physicians' Record Company.

Jenkins, T. (1988). New roles for nursing professionals. In M. J. Ball, K. J. Hannah, U. Gerdin Jelger, & H. Peterson (Eds.), *Nursing informatics: Where caring and technology meet.* New York: Springer, pp. 88–95.

Kraemer, K. S., Dickhoven, S., et al. (1987). *Datawars: The political modeling on federal policymaking.* New York: Columbia University Press.

LaDuke, S. (2000). NIC puts nursing into words: a common language empowers nurses to describe, validate, and control their practice. *Nursing Management, 31* (7), 43–44.

McCloskey, J. C. (1981). Nursing care plans and problem-oriented health records. In H. H. Werley and M. R. Grier (Eds.), *Nursing information systems.* New York: Springer, pp. 120–142.

McCloskey, J. C., & Bulechek, G. M. (1992). Intervention schemes. In *Papers from the Nursing Minimum Data Set Conference.* Edmonton, Alberta: Canadian Nurses Association, pp. 77–91.

McCloskey, J. C., Bulechek, G. M., & Tripp-Reimer, T. (1995). Response to Cody. *Nursing Outlook, 43* (2), 93–94.

McCormick, K. A., & Jones, C. B. (1998, September 30). Is one taxonomy needed for health care vocabularies and classifications? *Online Journal of Issues in Nursing.* Available: http://www.nursingworld.org/ojin/tpc7/tpc7_2 htm

Martin, K. S. & Scheet, N. (1992). *The Omaha System: Applications for community health nursing.* Philadelphia: W. B. Saunders.

Star, S. L., & Strauss, A. (1999). Layers of silence, arenas of voice: The ecology of visible and invisible work. *Computer Supported Cooperative Work: The Journal of Collaborative Computing* 8 (1/2), 9–30.

Tripp-Reimer, T., Woodworth, G., McCloskey, G., & Bulechek, G. (1996). The dimensional structure of nursing interventions. *Nursing Research, 45,* 10–17.

Zielstorff, R. D., Hudgings, C. I. Grobe, S. J., & The National Commission on Nursing Implementation Project (NCNIP) Task Force on Nursing Information Systems. (1993). *Next-generation nursing information systems: Essential characteristics for professional practice.* Washington, DC: American Nurses Publishing.

Conclusion: 5
The Benefits of a Unified Classification

Joanne McCloskey Dochterman
and Dorothy Jones

This monograph focuses on the effort to develop a common organizing structure (taxonomy) for harmonization of NANDA diagnoses, NIC interventions, and NOC outcomes. The structure itself appears as Table 2-6 (see Chapter 2, page 20), entitled Taxonomy of Nursing Practice. It is a good first effort toward providing a means to organize diagnoses, interventions, and outcomes in the same way. Having a common structure is more efficient than having separate structures and facilitates implementation of all the languages in practice and education. The proposed structure is placed in the public domain so that developers of other classifications and various other users can have easy access. The developers of NANDA, NIC, and NOC are committed to placing their diagnoses, interventions, and outcomes in the structure and to disseminating this in forthcoming publications. Future discussions of the issues involved in various placements will assist in refining the structure. The long-range goal is to achieve one unified classification consisting of diagnoses, interventions, and outcomes organized within the same structure.

Many groups may benefit from having a common unified nursing language classification, including educators, clinicians, researchers, and administrators. Informatics specialists will also be able to integrate a common unified classification of nursing language in the development of information systems that can be improved from refinement, accuracy, and clarity of terms used to communicate nursing to others. Some of the advantages for a common structure were listed in Chapter 2; the advantages and uses are further defined here so that readers of this monograph will be able to more readily implement the knowledge gained.

Education

Educators have long been concerned with the effectiveness and overall utility of teaching students different classification systems for communicating nursing diagnoses, interventions, and outcomes. The proposed unified nursing classification system will

- Help define essential content for nursing practice at the undergraduate and graduate levels.
- Provide a structure for curriculum design.
- Support the continued teaching of clinical judgment and critical thinking within the nursing curriculum.
- Enable faculty to focus on teaching one classification system.
- Increase student ease with documenting, especially within the proposed standardized electronic patient record.
- Provide a focus for research and clinical investigations by student researchers.
- Foster the integration of nursing theory to guide clinical practice.
- Increase opportunities for concept development, analysis, and evaluation in graduate courses, advancing both language and knowledge development
- Assist educators in linking knowledge with clinical practice.

Clinical Practice

Within the current healthcare environment, clinicians are searching for ways to accurately document care comprehensively, efficiently, in a timely way, and accurately. Stressors in the workplace and the impact of decreased resources challenge the nurse and often compromise documentation. The use of a unifying nursing classification will help clinicians

- Improve documentation by providing a structure for nurses to describe the patient experience more accurately.
- Identify nursing contributions to patient care outcomes more efficiently and effectively.
- Increase the use of language to articulate practice to consumers, other healthcare providers, administrators, and policy makers.
- Promote the use of the content addressed in the proposed unifying NNN structure as essential content for evidence-based practice.
- Create movement toward a culturally sensitive, standardized nursing assessment framework to evaluate function.
- Provide support for the use of all three dimensions of clinical reasoning, including assessment data used to make a clinical judgment, the diagnoses linked to outcome measures, and nursing actions used to resolve the problem.
- Help articulate concepts such as complexity and differentiated practice more accurately and with sensitivity to provider knowledge and experience.

Research and Knowledge Development

As nursing grows as a science, it will be important to articulate the content of the discipline and describe the patient problems solved by the nurse giving care.

The development of a common unifying nursing language can facilitate knowledge development and promote research initiatives that develop, test, and refine knowledge. This will result in

▌ Continued development and refinement of concepts and content essential to the discipline of nursing and language development.
▌ Development of midrange theories that can guide practice and be linked to the clinical judgment process within nursing.
▌ Use of new research methodologies that test and refine existing nursing language.
▌ Generation of research initiatives to identify high-incidence patient problems within and across settings.
▌ Evaluating patient outcomes that are linked to diagnosis and intervention strategies.
▌ Establishment of outcome indicators described by using nursing language.
▌ Defining essential content for nursing practice at the undergraduate and graduate levels.
▌ Development, testing, and evaluation of predictive models that can be used to respond to the patient experience with quality cost-effective care strategies.
▌ Analyzing an extensive, available database that can more accurately examine the effectiveness of nursing's contributions to patient care.

Administration

Nurse administrators will benefit from the use of a common unified classification of nursing language in multiple ways. These include, but are not limited to:

▌ Improved documentation of nursing care across patient populations and settings critical to meeting standards used in clinical organizational evaluation.
▌ Participating in the development and purchase of information systems and defining the content needed to capture nursing practice particularly in the electronic patient medical record information (PMRI).
▌ Standardization of nursing data that can be analyzed and further researched by more accurate costing out services.
▌ Accurately informing the development of a reimbursement system for nursing services within the organization's infrastructure.
▌ Identification of common nursing problems, patient co-morbidity, and the mix of staff needed to address patient problems in a quality, cost-effective manner.
▌ Use of nursing diagnoses, interventions, and outcomes to communicate and substantiate the contributions of nursing to policy makers and hospital administrators.
▌ Describing a practice environment that is patient focused and grounded in nursing inquiry and knowledge needed to identify, explain, and effect patient responses in health and illness.

These lists of various uses demonstrate the importance of harmonization. We believe that the publication of this monograph represents an important step forward in the ongoing efforts of many individuals in the United States and other countries to describe, document, and study the contributions of nursing care. Although the Taxonomy of Nursing Practice structure may not be a perfect fit for all concepts from differing classifications, it represents a good beginning effort in effecting a harmonization of previous work in this area.

Glossary of Terms | A

Class—The second level of the taxonomy, less abstract than the top domain level, in which the concepts (diagnoses, interventions or outcomes) are grouped.

Classification—The ordering or arranging of items (e.g. defining characteristics, activities, indicators) based on relationships, and assignment of names (e.g. diagnoses, interventions, outcomes) to the groups of items.

Diagnoses—Clinical judgments about individual, family, or community responses to actual or potential problems/life processes that provide the basis for selection of nursing interventions to achieve outcomes for which the nurse is accountable (NANDA).

Domain—The top, most abstract level of a taxonomy.

Interventions—Treatments performed based upon clinical judgment and knowledge to enhance patient outcomes (NIC).

Organizing Structure/Unifying Structure/Taxonomic Structure—A way to group concepts based upon similarities; terms are used interchangeably.

Outcomes—Measurable individual, family, or community states, behaviors or perceptions largely influenced by and responsive to nursing interventions (NOC).

Standardized Language—Agreed-upon labels and definitions for concepts that are not changed unless the change is approved in a formal review process and officially published.

Taxonomy—A systematic organization of concepts based upon similarities and into what can be considered a conceptual framework; differs from the taxonomic structure in that it contains the structure plus the placement of concepts.

Terminology—Words for concepts, the vocabulary; sometimes used interchangeably with classification.

NANDA Diagnosis Labels and Definitions
(155 Diagnoses)

B

Activity Intolerance
Insufficient physiological or psychological energy to endure or complete required or desired daily activities

Activity Intolerance, Risk for
At risk for experiencing insufficient physiological or psychological energy to endure or complete required or desired daily activities

Adjustment, Impaired
Inability to modify lifestyle/behavior in a manner consistent with a change in health status

Airway Clearance, Ineffective
Inability to clear secretions or obstructions from the respiratory tract to maintain a clear airway

Anxiety
Vague uneasy feeling of discomfort or dread accompanied by an autonomic response (the source often nonspecific or unknown to the individual); a feeling of apprehension caused by anticipation of danger. It is an alerting signal that warns of impending danger and enables the individual to take measures to deal with threat.

Aspiration, Risk for
At risk for entry of gastrointestinal secretions, oropharyngeal secretions, solids, or fluids into tracheobronchial passages

Autonomic Dysreflexia
Life-threatening, uninhibited sympathetic response of the nervous system to a noxious stimulus after a spinal cord injury at T7 or above.

Autonomic Dysreflexia, Risk for
At risk for life-threatening, uninhibited response of the sympathetic nervous system, post spinal shock, in an individual with spinal cord injury or lesion at T6 or above (has been demonstrated in patients with injuries at T7 and T8).

Source: *NANDA Nursing Diagnosis: Definitions and Classification 2001–2002* (Philadelphia: NANDA). Reproduced with permission of NANDA International, 1211 Locust Street, Philadelphia, PA 19107, 215-545-8105.

Body Image, Disturbed
Confusion in mental picture of one's physical self

Body Temperature, Risk for Imbalanced
At risk for failure to maintain body temperature within normal range

Bowel Incontinence
Change in normal bowel habits characterized by involuntary passage of stool

Breastfeeding, Effective
Mother-infant dyad/family exhibits adequate proficiency and satisfaction with breastfeeding process

Breastfeeding, Ineffective
Dissatisfaction or difficulty a mother, infant, or child experiences with the breastfeeding process

Breastfeeding, Interrupted
Break in the continuity of the breastfeeding process as a result of inability or inadvisability to put baby to breast for feeding

Breathing Pattern, Ineffective
Inspiration and/or expiration that does not provide adequate ventilation

Cardiac Output, Decreased
Inadequate blood pumped by the heart to meet metabolic demands of the body

Caregiver Role Strain
Difficulty in performing caregiver role

Caregiver Role Strain, Risk for
Caregiver is vulnerable for felt difficulty in performing the family caregiver role

Communication, Impaired Verbal
Decreased, delayed, or absent ability to receive, process, transmit, and use a system of symbols

Community Coping, Ineffective
Pattern of community activities (for adaptation and problem solving) that is unsatisfactory for meeting the demands or needs of the community

Community Coping, Readiness for Enhanced
Pattern of community activities for adaptation and problem solving that is satisfactory for meeting the demands or needs of the community but can be improved for management of current and future problems/stressors

Community Therapeutic Regimen Management, Ineffective
Pattern of regulating and integrating into community processes programs for treatment of illness and the sequelae of illness that are unsatisfactory for meeting health-related goals

Confusion, Acute
The abrupt onset of a cluster of global, transient changes and disturbances in attention, cognition, psychomotor activity, level of consciousness, and/or sleep/wake cycle

Confusion, Chronic
Irreversible, long-standing, and/or progressive deterioration of intellect and personality characterized by decreased ability to interpret environmental stimuli; decreased capacity for intellectual thought processes; and manifested by disturbances of memory, orientation, and behavior

Constipation
Decrease in a person's normal frequency of defecation accompanied by difficult or incomplete passage of stool and/or passage of excessively hard, dry stools

Constipation, Perceived
Self-diagnosis of constipation and abuse of laxatives, enemas, and suppositories to ensure a daily bowel movement

Constipation, Risk for
At risk for a decrease in normal frequency of defecation accompanied by difficult or incomplete passage of stool and/or passage of excessive hard, dry stool

Coping, Defensive
Repeated projection of falsely positive self-evaluation based on a self-protective pattern that defends against underlying perceived threats to positive self-regard

Coping, Ineffective
Inability to form a valid appraisal of the stressors, inadequate choices of practiced responses, and/or inability to use available resources

Death Anxiety
Apprehension, worry, or fear related to death or dying

Decisional Conflict (Specify)
Uncertainty about course of action to be taken when choice among competing actions involves risk, loss, or challenge to personal life values

Denial, Ineffective
Conscious or unconscious attempt to disavow the knowledge or meaning of an event to reduce anxiety/fear but leading to the detriment of health

Dentition, Impaired
Disruption in tooth development/eruption patterns or structural integrity of individual teeth

Development, Risk for Delayed
At risk for delay of 25% or more in one or more of the areas of social or self-regulatory behavior, or in cognitive, language, gross or fine motor skills

Diarrhea
Passage of loose, unformed stools

Disuse Syndrome, Risk for
At risk for deterioration of body systems as the result of prescribed or unavoidable musculoskeletal inactivity

Diversional Activity, Deficient
Decreased stimulation from (or interest or engagement in) recreational or leisure activities

Energy Field, Disturbed
Disruption in the flow of energy surrounding a person's being that results in a disharmony of the body, mind, and/or spirit

Environmental Interpretation Syndrome, Impaired
Consistent lack of orientation to person, place, time, or circumstances over more than three to six months necessitating a protective environment

Failure to Thrive, Adult
Progressive functional deterioration of a physical and cognitive nature. The individual's ability to live with multisystem diseases, cope with ensuing problems, and manage his/her care are remarkably diminished.

Falls, Risk for
Increased susceptibility to falling that may cause physical harm

Family Coping, Compromised
Usually supportive primary person (family member or close friend) provides insufficient, ineffective, or compromised support, comfort, assistance, or encouragement that the client may need to manage or master adaptive tasks related to his/her health challenge

Family Coping, Disabled
Behavior of significant person (family member or other primary person) that disables his/her own capacities and the client's capacities to effectively address tasks essential to either person's adaptation to the health challenge

Family Coping, Readiness for Enhanced
Effective management of adaptive tasks by family member involved with the client's health challenge, who now exhibits desire and readiness for enhanced health and growth in regard to self and in relation to the client

Family Processes, Dysfunctional: Alcoholism
Psychosocial, spiritual, and physiological functions of the family unit are chronically disorganized, which leads to conflict, denial of problems, resistance to change, ineffective problem solving, and a series of self-perpetuating crises

Family Processes, Interrupted
Change in family relationships and/or functioning

Family Therapeutic Regimen Management, Ineffective
Pattern of regulating and integrating into daily living a program for treatment of illness and the sequelae of illness that is unsatisfactory for meeting specific health goals

Fatigue
An overwhelming sustained sense of exhaustion and decreased capacity for physical and mental work at usual level

Fear
Response to perceived threat that is consciously recognized as a danger

Fluid Volume, Deficient
Decreased intravascular, interstitial, and/or intracellular fluid. This refers to dehydration water loss alone without change in sodium

Fluid Volume, Excess
Increased isotonic fluid retention

Fluid Volume, Risk for Deficient
At risk of experiencing vascular, cellular, or intracellular dehydration

Fluid Volume, Risk for Imbalanced
At risk for a decrease, increase, or rapid shift from one to the other of intravascular, interstitial, and/or intracellular fluid. This refers to body fluid loss, gain, or both.

Gas Exchange, Impaired
Excess or deficit in oxygenation and/or carbon dioxide elimination at the alveolar-capillary membrane

Grieving, Anticipatory
Intellectual and emotional responses and behaviors by which individuals, families, and communities work through the process of modifying self-concept based on the perception of potential loss

Grieving, Dysfunctional
Extended, unsuccessful use of intellectual and emotional responses by which individuals, families, and communities attempt to work through the process of modifying self-concept based on the perception of loss

Growth and Development, Delayed
Deviations from age-group norms

Growth, Risk for Disproportionate
At risk for growth above the 97th percentile or below the 3rd percentile for age, crossing two percentile channels; disproportionate growth

Health Maintenance, Ineffective
Inability to identify, manage and/or seek out help to maintain health

Health-Seeking Behaviors (Specify)
Active seeking (by a person in stable health) of ways to alter personal health habits and/or the environment in order to move toward a higher level of health

Home Maintenance, Impaired
Inability to independently maintain a safe growth-promoting immediate environment

Hopelessness
Subjective state in which an individual sees limited or no alternatives or personal choices available and is unable to mobilize energy on own behalf

Hyperthermia
Body temperature elevated above normal range

Hypothermia
Body temperature below normal range

Infant Behavior, Disorganized
Disintegrated physiological and neurobehavioral response to the environment

Infant Behavior, Risk for Disorganized
Risk for alteration in integration and modulation of the physiological and behavioral systems of functioning (i.e., autonomic, motor, state, organizational, self-regulatory, and attentional-interactional systems)

Infant Behavior: Organized, Readiness for Enhanced
A pattern of modulation of the physiologic and behavioral systems of functioning of an infant (i.e., autonomic, motor, state, organizational, self-regulatory, and attentional-interactional systems) that is satisfactory but that can be improved, resulting in higher levels of integration in response to environmental stimuli

Infant Feeding Pattern, Ineffective
Impaired ability to suck or coordinate the suck-swallow response

Infection, Risk for
At increased risk for being invaded by pathogenic organisms

Injury, Risk for
At risk of injury as a result of environmental conditions interacting with the individual's adaptive and defensive resources

Intracranial Adaptive Capacity, Decreased
Intracranial fluid dynamic mechanisms that normally compensate for increases in intracranial volumes are compromised, resulting in repeated disproportionate increases in intracranial pressure (ICP) in response to a variety of noxious and non-noxious stimuli

Knowledge, Deficient (Specify)
Absence or deficiency of cognitive information related to specific topic

Latex Allergy Response
An allergic response to natural latex rubber products

Latex Allergy Response, Risk for
At risk for allergic response to natural latex rubber products

Loneliness, Risk for
At risk of experiencing vague dysphoria

Memory, Impaired
Inability to remember or recall bits of information or behavioral skills. (Impaired memory may be attributed to pathophysiological or situational causes that are either temporary or permanent)

Mobility: Bed, Impaired
Limitation of independent movement from one bed position to another

Mobility: Physical, Impaired
Limitation in independent, purposeful physical movement of the body or of one or more extremities

Mobility: Wheelchair, Impaired
Limitation of independent operation of wheelchair within environment

Nausea
Unpleasant, wavelike sensation in the back of the throat, epigastrium, or throughout the abdomen that may or may not lead to vomiting

Noncompliance
Behavior of person and/or caregiver that fails to coincide with a health-promoting or therapeutic plan agreed upon by the person (and/or family, and/or community) and healthcare professional. In the presence of an agreed upon health-promoting or therapeutic plan, person's or caregiver's behavior may be fully or partially nonadherent and may lead to clinically effective, partially ineffective outcomes.

Nutrition: Imbalanced, Less Than Body Requirements
Intake of nutrients insufficient to meet metabolic needs

Nutrition: Imbalanced, More Than Body Requirements
Intake of nutrients that exceeds metabolic needs

Nutrition: Imbalanced, Risk for More Than Body Requirements
At risk for an intake of nutrients that exceeds metabolic needs

Oral Mucous Membrane, Impaired
Disruption of the lips and soft tissue of the oral cavity

Pain, Acute
Unpleasant sensory and emotional experience arising from actual or potential tissue damage or described in terms of such damage (International Association for the Study of Pain); sudden or slow onset of any intensity from mild to severe with an anticipated or predictable end and a duration of less than six months

Pain, Chronic
Unpleasant sensory and emotional experience arising from actual or potential tissue damage or described in terms of such damage (International Association for the Study of Pain); sudden or slow onset of any intensity from mild to severe, constant or recurring without an anticipated or predictable end and a duration of greater than six months

Parent/Infant/Child Attachment, Risk for Impaired
Disruption of the interactive process between parent/significant other and infant that fosters the development of a protective and nurturing reciprocal relationship

Parental Role Conflict
Parent experience of role confusion and conflict in response to crisis

Parenting, Impaired
Inability of the primary caretaker to create, maintain, or regain an environment that promotes the optimum growth and development of the child

Parenting, Risk for Impaired
Risk for inability of the primary caretaker to create, maintain, or regain an environment that promotes the optimum growth and development of the child

Perioperative Positioning Injury, Risk for
At risk for injury as a result of the environmental conditions found in the perioperative setting

Peripheral Neurovascular Dysfunction, Risk for
At risk for disruption in circulation, sensation, or motion of an extremity

Personal Identity, Disturbed
Inability to distinguish between self and nonself

Poisoning, Risk for
At accentuated risk of accidental exposure to, or ingestion of, drugs or dangerous products in doses sufficient to cause poisoning

Post-Trauma Syndrome
Sustained maladaptative response to a traumatic, overwhelming event

Post-Trauma Syndrome, Risk for
At risk for sustained maladaptive response to traumatic, overwhelming event

Powerlessness
Perception that one's own action will not significantly affect an outcome; a perceived lack of control over a current situation or immediate happening

Powerlessness, Risk for
At risk for perceived lack of control over a situation and/or one's ability to significantly affect an outcome

Protection, Ineffective
Decrease in the ability to guard self from internal or external threats such as illness or injury

Rape-Trauma Syndrome
Sustained maladaptive response to a forced, violent sexual penetration against the victim's will and consent

Rape-Trauma Syndrome: Compound Reaction
Forced violent sexual penetration against the victim's will and consent. The trauma syndrome that develops from this attack or attempted attack includes an acute phase of disorganization of the victim's lifestyle and a long-term process of reorganization of lifestyle.

Rape-Trauma Syndrome: Silent Reaction
Forced violent sexual penetration against the victim's will and consent. The trauma syndrome that develops from this attack or attempted attack includes an acute phase of disorganization of the victim's lifestyle and a long-term process of reorganization of lifestyle.

Relocation Stress Syndrome
Physiological and/or psychosocial disturbance following transfer from one environment to another

Relocation Stress Syndrome, Risk for
At risk for physiological and/or psychosocial disturbance following transfer from one environment to another

Role Performance, Ineffective
Patterns of behavior and self-expression that do not match the environmental context, norms, and expectations

Self-Care Deficit: Bathing/Hygiene
Impaired ability to perform or complete bathing/hygiene activities for oneself

Self-Care Deficit: Dressing/Grooming
Impaired ability to perform or complete dressing and grooming activities for self

Self-Care Deficit: Feeding
Impaired ability to perform or complete feeding activities

Self-Care Deficit: Toileting
Impaired ability to perform or complete own toileting activities

Self-Esteem: Chronic Low
Long-standing negative self-evaluation/feelings about self or self-capabilities

Self-Esteem: Situational Low
Development of a negative perception of self-worth in response to a current situation (specify)

Self-Esteem: Situational Low, Risk for
At risk for developing negative perception of self-worth in response to a current situation (specify)

Self-Mutilation
Deliberate self-injurious behavior causing tissue damage with the intent of causing nonfatal injury to attain relief of tension

Self-Mutilation, Risk for
At risk for deliberate self-injurious behavior causing tissue damage with the intent of causing nonfatal injury to attain relief of tension

Sensory Perception, Disturbed (Specify: Visual, Auditory, Kinesthetic, Gustatory, Tactile, Olfactory)
Change in the amount or patterning of incoming stimuli accompanied by a diminished, exaggerated, distorted, or impaired response to such stimuli

Sexual Dysfunction
Change in sexual function that is viewed as unsatisfying, unrewarding, inadequate

Sexuality Patterns, Ineffective
Expressions of concern regarding own sexuality

Skin Integrity, Impaired
Altered epidermis and/or dermis

Skin Integrity, Risk for Impaired
At risk for skin being adversely altered

Sleep Deprivation
Prolonged periods of time without sleep (sustained natural, periodic suspension of relative consciousness)

Sleep Pattern, Disturbed
Time-limited disruption of sleep (natural, periodic suspension of consciousness) amount and quality

Social Interaction, Impaired
Insufficient or excessive quantity or ineffective quality of social exchange

Social Isolation
Aloneness experienced by the individual and perceived as imposed by others and as a negative or threatening state

Sorrow: Chronic
Cyclical, recurring, and potentially progressive pattern of pervasive sadness experienced (by a parent, caregiver, individual with chronic illness or disability) in response to continual loss, throughout the trajectory of an illness or disability

Spiritual Distress
Disruption in the life principle that pervades a person's entire being and that integrates and transcends one's biological and psychosocial nature

Spiritual Distress, Risk for
At risk for an altered sense of harmonious connectedness with all of life and the universe in which dimensions that transcend and empower the self may be disrupted

Spiritual Well-Being, Readiness for Enhanced
Process of developing/unfolding of mystery through harmonious interconnectedness that springs from inner strengths

Suffocation, Risk for
Accentuated risk of accidental suffocation (inadequate air available for inhalation)

Suicide, Risk for
At risk for self-inflicted, life-threatening injury

Surgical Recovery, Delayed
Extension of the number of postoperative days required to initiate and perform activities that maintain life, health, and well-being

Swallowing, Impaired
Abnormal functioning of the swallowing mechanism associated with deficits in oral, pharyngeal, or esophageal structure or function

Therapeutic Regimen Management, Effective
Pattern of regulating and integrating into daily living a program for treatment of illness and its sequelae that is satisfactory for meeting specific health goals

Therapeutic Regimen Management, Ineffective
Pattern of regulating and integrating into daily living a program for treatment of illness and the sequelae of illness that is unsatisfactory for meeting specific health goals

Thermoregulation, Ineffective
Temperature fluctuation between hypothermia and hyperthermia

Thought Processes, Disturbed
Disruption in cognitive operations and activities

Tissue Integrity, Impaired
Damage to mucous membrane, corneal, integumentary, or subcutaneous tissues

Tissue Perfusion, Ineffective (Specify Type: Renal, Cerebral, Cardiopulmonary, Gastro-intestinal, Peripheral)
Decrease in oxygen resulting in the failure to nourish the tissues at the capillary level

Transfer Ability, Impaired
Limitation of independent movement between two nearby surfaces

Trauma, Risk for
Accentuated risk of accidental tissue injury (e.g., wound, burn, fracture)

Unilateral Neglect
Lack of awareness and attention to one side of the body

Urinary Elimination, Impaired
Disturbance in urine elimination

Urinary Incontinence: Functional
Inability of usually continent person to reach toilet in time to avoid unintentional loss of urine

Urinary Incontinence: Reflex
Involuntary loss of urine at somewhat predictable intervals when a specific bladder volume is reached

Urinary Incontinence: Stress
Loss of less than 50 ml of urine occurring with increased abdominal pressure

Urinary Incontinence: Total
Continuous and unpredictable loss of urine

Urinary Incontinence: Urge
Involuntary passage of urine occurring soon after a strong sense of urgency to void

Urinary Incontinence: Urge, Risk for
At risk for involuntary loss of urine associated with a sudden, strong sensation or urinary urgency

Urinary Retention
Incomplete emptying of the bladder

Ventilation, Impaired Spontaneous
Decreased energy reserves result in an individual's inability to maintain breathing adequate to support life

Ventilatory Weaning Response, Dysfunctional
Inability to adjust to lowered levels of mechanical ventilator support that interrupts and prolongs the weaning process

Violence: Other-Directed, Risk for
At risk for behaviors in which an individual demonstrates that he/she can be physically, emotionally, and/or sexually harmful to others

Violence: Self-Directed, Risk for
At risk for behaviors in which an individual demonstrates that he/she can be physically, emotionally, and/or sexually harmful to self

Walking, Impaired
Limitation of independent movement within the environment on foot

Wandering
Meandering, aimless, or repetitive locomotion that exposes the individual to harm; frequently incongruent with boundaries, limits, or obstacles

NIC Intervention Labels and Definitions ($n = 486$)

C

Numbers are unique intervention codes related to placement in taxonomic structure.

6400   Abuse Protection Support
Identification of high-risk dependent relationships and actions to prevent further infliction of physical or emotional harm

6402   Abuse Protection Support: Child
Identification of high-risk, dependent child relationships and actions to prevent possible or further infliction of physical, sexual, or emotional harm or neglect of basic necessities of life

6403   Abuse Protection Support: Domestic Partner
Identification of high-risk, dependent domestic relationships and actions to prevent possible or further infliction of physical, sexual, or emotional harm or exploitation of a domestic partner

6404   Abuse Protection Support: Elder
Identification of high-risk, dependent elder relationships and actions to prevent possible or further infliction of physical, sexual, or emotional harm; neglect of basic necessities of life; or exploitation

6408   Abuse Protection Support: Religious
Identification of high-risk, controlling religious relationships and actions to prevent infliction of physical, sexual, or emotional harm and/or exploitation

1910   Acid-Base Management
Promotion of acid-base balance and prevention of complications resulting from acid-base imbalance

1911   Acid-Base Management: Metabolic Acidosis
Promotion of acid-base balance and prevention of complications resulting from serum HCO_3 levels lower than desired

Source: McCloskey, J.C., & Bulechek, G.B. (Eds.). (2000). *Nursing Interventions Classification (NIC), 3rd ed.* St. Louis: Mosby, Inc. Reproduced with permission of the publisher.

1912   Acid-Base Management: Metabolic Alkalosis
Promotion of acid-base balance and prevention of complications resulting from serum HCO_3 levels higher than desired

1913   Acid-Base Management: Respiratory Acidosis
Promotion of acid-base balance and prevention of complications resulting from serum PCO_2 levels higher than desired

1914   Acid-Base Management: Respiratory Alkalosis
Promotion of acid-base balance and prevention of complications resulting from serum PCO_2 levels lower than desired

1920   Acid-Base Monitoring
Collection and analysis of patient data to regulate acid-base balance

4920   Active Listening
Attending closely to and attaching significance to a patient's verbal and nonverbal messages

4310   Activity Therapy
Prescription of and assistance with specific physical, cognitive, social, and spiritual activities to increase the range, frequency, or duration of an individual's (or group's) activity

1320   Acupressure
Application of firm, sustained pressure to special points on the body to decrease pain, produce relaxation, and prevent or reduce nausea

7310   Admission Care
Facilitating entry of a patient into a healthcare facility

3120   Airway Insertion and Stabilization
Insertion or assisting with insertion and stabilization of an artificial airway

3140   Airway Management
Facilitation of patency of air passages

3160   Airway Suctioning
Removal of airway secretions by inserting a suction catheter into the patient's oral airway and/or trachea

6410   Allergy Management
Identification, treatment, and prevention of allergic responses to food, medications, insect bites, contrast material, blood, or other substances

6700   Amnioinfusion
Infusion of fluid into the uterus during labor to relieve umbilical cord compression or to dilute meconium-stained fluid

3420   Amputation Care
Promotion of physical and psychological healing after amputation of a body part

2210   Analgesic Administration
Use of pharmacologic agents to reduce or eliminate pain

2214   Analgesic Administration: Intraspinal
Administration of pharmacologic agents into the epidural or intrathecal space to reduce or eliminate pain

6412   Anaphylaxis Management
Promotion of adequate ventilation and tissue perfusion for a patient with a severe allergic (antigen-antibody) reaction

2840   Anesthesia Administration
Preparation for and administration of anesthetic agents and monitoring of patient responsiveness during administration

4640   Anger Control Assistance
Facilitation of the expression of anger in an adaptive nonviolent manner

4320   Animal-Assisted Therapy
Purposeful use of animals to provide affection, attention, diversion, and relaxation

5210   Anticipatory Guidance
Preparation of patient for an anticipated developmental and/or situational crisis

5820   Anxiety Reduction
Minimizing apprehension, dread, foreboding, or uneasiness related to an unidentified source of anticipated danger

6420   Area Restriction
Limitation of patient mobility to a specified area for purposes of safety or behavior management

4330   Art Therapy
Facilitation of communication through drawings or other art forms

3180   Artificial Airway Management
Maintenance of endotracheal and tracheostomy tubes and preventing complications associated with their use

3200   Aspiration Precautions
Prevention or minimization of risk factors in the patient at risk for aspiration

4340   Assertiveness Training
Assistance with the effective expression of feelings, needs, and ideas while respecting the rights of others

6710   Attachment Promotion
Facilitation of the development of the parent–infant relationship

5840   Autogenic Training
Assisting with self-suggestions about feelings of heaviness and warmth for the purpose of inducing relaxation

2860   Autotransfusion
Collecting and reinfusing blood that has been lost intraoperatively or postoperatively from clean wounds

1610   Bathing
Cleaning of the body for the purposes of relaxation, cleanliness, and healing

0740　Bed Rest Care
Promotion of comfort and safety and prevention of complications for a patient unable to get out of bed

7610　Bedside Laboratory Testing
Performance of laboratory tests at the bedside or point of care

4350　Behavior Management
Helping a patient to manage negative behavior

4352　Behavior Management: Overactivity/Inattention
Provision of a therapeutic milieu that safely accommodates the patient's attention deficit and/or overactivity while promoting optimal function

4354　Behavior Management: Self-Harm
Assisting the patient to decrease or eliminate self-mutilating or self-abusive behaviors

4356　Behavior Management: Sexual
Delineation and prevention of socially unacceptable sexual behaviors

4360　Behavior Modification
Promotion of a behavior change

4362　Behavior Modification: Social Skills
Assisting the patient to develop or improve interpersonal social skills

4680　Bibliotherapy
Use of literature to enhance the expression of feelings and the gaining of insight

5860　Biofeedback
Assisting the patient to modify a body function using feedback from instrumentation

6720　Birthing
Delivery of a baby

0550　Bladder Irrigation
Instillation of a solution into the bladder to provide cleansing or medication

4010　Bleeding Precautions
Reduction of stimuli that may induce bleeding or hemorrhage in at-risk patients

4020　Bleeding Reduction
Limitation of the loss of blood volume during an episode of bleeding

4021　Bleeding Reduction: Antepartum Uterus
Limitation of the amount of blood loss from the pregnant uterus during third trimester of pregnancy

4022　Bleeding Reduction: Gastrointestinal
Limitation of the amount of blood loss from the upper and lower gastrointestinal tract and related complications

4024　Bleeding Reduction: Nasal
Limitation of the amount of blood loss from the nasal cavity

4026   Bleeding Reduction: Postpartum Uterus
Limitation of the amount of blood loss from the postpartum uterus

4028   Bleeding Reduction: Wound
Limitation of the blood loss from a wound that may be a result of trauma, incisions, or placement of a tube or catheter

4030   Blood Products Administration
Administration of blood or blood products and monitoring of patient's response

5220   Body Image Enhancement
Improving a patient's conscious and unconscious perceptions and attitudes toward his/her body

0140   Body Mechanics Promotion
Facilitating the use of posture and movement in daily activities to prevent fatigue and musculoskeletal strain or injury

1052   Bottle Feeding
Preparation and administration of fluids to an infant via a bottle

0410   Bowel Incontinence Care
Promotion of bowel continence and maintenance of perianal skin integrity

0412   Bowel Incontinence Care: Encopresis
Promotion of bowel continence in children

0420   Bowel Irrigation
Instillation of a substance into the lower gastrointestinal tract

0430   Bowel Management
Establishment and maintenance of a regular pattern of bowel elimination

0440   Bowel Training
Assisting the patient to train the bowel to evacuate at specific intervals

6522   Breast Examination
Inspection and palpation of the breasts and related areas

1054   Breastfeeding Assistance
Preparing a new mother to breastfeed her infant

5880   Calming Technique
Reducing anxiety in patient experiencing acute distress

4040   Cardiac Care
Limitation of complications resulting from an imbalance between myocardial oxygen supply and demand for a patient with symptoms of impaired cardiac function

4044   Cardiac Care: Acute
Limitation of complications for a patient recently experiencing an episode of an imbalance between myocardial oxygen supply and demand resulting in impaired cardiac function

4046   Cardiac Care: Rehabilitative
Promotion of maximum functional activity level for a patient who has suffered an episode of impaired cardiac function which resulted from an imbalance between myocardial oxygen supply and demand

4050   Cardiac Precautions
Prevention of an acute episode of impaired cardiac function by minimizing myocardial oxygen consumption or increasing myocardial oxygen supply

7040   Caregiver Support
Provision of the necessary information, advocacy, and support to facilitate primary patient care by someone other than a healthcare professional

7320   Case Management
Coordinating care and advocating for specified individuals and patient populations across settings to reduce cost, reduce resource use, improve quality of health care, and achieve desired outcomes

0762   Cast Care: Maintenance
Care of a cast after the drying period

0764   Cast Care: Wet
Care of a new cast during the drying period

2540   Cerebral Edema Management
Limitation of secondary cerebral injury resulting from swelling of brain tissue

2550   Cerebral Perfusion Promotion
Promotion of adequate perfusion and limitation of complications for a patient experiencing or at risk for inadequate cerebral perfusion

6750   Cesarean Section Care
Preparation and support of patient delivering a baby by cesarean section

2240   Chemotherapy Management
Assisting the patient and family to understand the action and minimize side effects of antineoplastic agents

3230   Chest Physiotherapy
Assisting the patient to move airway secretions from peripheral airways to more central airways for expectoration and/or suctioning

6760   Childbirth Preparation
Providing information and support to facilitate childbirth and to enhance the ability of an individual to develop and perform the role of parent

4062   Circulatory Care: Arterial Insufficiency
Promotion of arterial circulation

4064   Circulatory Care: Mechanical Assist Device
Temporary support of the circulation through the use of mechanical devices or pumps

4066   Circulatory Care: Venous Insufficiency
Promotion of venous circulation

4070   Circulatory Precautions
Protection of a localized area with limited perfusion

6140   Code Management
Coordination of emergency measures to sustain life

4700 Cognitive Restructuring

Challenging a patient to alter distorted thought patterns and view self and the world more realistically

4720 Cognitive Stimulation

Promotion of awareness and comprehension of surroundings by utilization of planned stimuli

8820 Communicable Disease Management

Working with a community to decrease and manage the incidence and prevalence of contagious diseases in a specific population

4974 Communication Enhancement: Hearing Deficit

Assistance in accepting and learning alternate methods for living with diminished hearing

4976 Communication Enhancement: Speech Deficit

Assistance in accepting and learning alternate methods for living with impaired speech

4978 Communication Enhancement: Visual Deficit

Assistance in accepting and learning alternate methods for living with diminished vision

8840 Community Disaster Preparedness

Preparing for an effective response to a large-scale disaster

8500 Community Health Development

Facilitating members of a community to identify a community's health concerns, mobilize resources, and implement solutions

5000 Complex Relationship Building

Establishing a therapeutic relationship with a patient who has difficulty interacting with others

5020 Conflict Mediation

Facilitation of constructive dialogue between opposing parties with a goal of resolving disputes in a mutually acceptable manner

2260 Conscious Sedation

Administration of sedatives, monitoring of the patient's response, and provision of necessary physiological support during a diagnostic or therapeutic procedure

0450 Constipation/Impaction Management

Prevention and alleviation of constipation/impaction

7910 Consultation

Using expert knowledge to work with those who seek help in problem-solving to enable individuals, families, groups, or agencies to achieve identified goals

1620 Contact Lens Care

Prevention of eye injury and lens damage by proper use of contact lenses

7620 Controlled Substance Checking

Promoting appropriate use and maintaining security of controlled substances

5230 Coping Enhancement

Assisting a patient to adapt to perceived stressors, changes, or threats that interfere with meeting life demands and roles

7630　Cost Containment
Management and facilitation of efficient and effective use of resources

3250　Cough Enhancement
Promotion of deep inhalation by the patient with subsequent generation of high intrathoracic pressures and compression of underlying lung parenchyma for the forceful expulsion of air

5240　Counseling
Use of an interactive helping process focusing on the needs, problems, or feelings of the patient and significant others to enhance or support coping, problem-solving, and interpersonal relationships

6160　Crisis Intervention
Use of short-term counseling to help the patient cope with a crisis and resume a state of functioning comparable to or better than the pre-crisis state

7640　Critical Path Development
Constructing and using a timed sequence of patient care activities to enhance desired patient outcomes in a cost-efficient manner

7330　Culture Brokerage
The deliberate use of culturally competent strategies to bridge or mediate between the patient's culture and the biomedical healthcare system

1340　Cutaneous Stimulation
Stimulation of the skin and underlying tissues for the purpose of decreasing undesirable signs and symptoms such as pain, muscle spasm, or inflammation

5250　Decision-Making Support
Providing information and support for a patient who is making a decision regarding health care

7650　Delegation
Transfer of responsibility for the performance of patient care while retaining accountability for the outcome

6440　Delirium Management
Provision of a safe and therapeutic environment for the patient who is experiencing an acute confusional state

6450　Delusion Management
Promoting the comfort, safety, and reality orientation of a patient experiencing false, fixed beliefs that have little or no basis in reality

6460　Dementia Management
Provision of a modified environment for the patient who is experiencing a chronic confusional state

8250　Developmental Care
Structuring the environment and providing care in response to the behavioral cues and states of the preterm infant

8272　Developmental Enhancement: Adolescent
Facilitating optimal physical, cognitive, social, and emotional growth of individuals during the transition from childhood to adulthood

8274 Developmental Enhancement: Child
Facilitating or teaching parents/caregivers to facilitate the optimal gross motor, fine motor, language, cognitive, social and emotional growth of preschool and school-age children

0460 Diarrhea Management
Prevention and alleviation of diarrhea

1020 Diet Staging
Instituting required diet restrictions with subsequent progression of diet as tolerated

7370 Discharge Planning
Preparation for moving a patient from one level of care to another within or outside the current health care agency

5900 Distraction
Purposeful focusing of attention away from undesirable sensations

7920 Documentation
Recording of pertinent patient data in a clinical record

1630 Dressing
Choosing, putting on, and removing clothes for a person who cannot do this for self

5260 Dying Care
Promotion of physical comfort and psychological peace in the final phase of life

2560 Dysreflexia Management
Prevention and elimination of stimuli that cause hyperactive reflexes and inappropriate autonomic responses in a patient with a cervical or high thoracic cord lesion

4090 Dysrhythmia Management
Preventing, recognizing, and facilitating treatment of abnormal cardiac rhythms

1640 Ear Care
Prevention or minimization of threats to ear or hearing

1030 Eating Disorders Management
Prevention and treatment of severe diet restriction and overexercising or binging and purging of food and fluids

2000 Electrolyte Management
Promotion of electrolyte balance and prevention of complications resulting from abnormal or undesired serum electrolyte levels

2001 Electrolyte Management: Hypercalcemia
Promotion of calcium balance and prevention of complications resulting from serum calcium levels higher than desired

2002 Electrolyte Management: Hyperkalemia
Promotion of potassium balance and prevention of complications resulting from serum potassium levels higher than desired

2003 Electrolyte Management: Hypermagnesemia
Promotion of magnesium balance and prevention of complications resulting from serum magnesium levels higher than desired

2004 Electrolyte Management: Hypernatremia
Promotion of sodium balance and prevention of complications resulting from serum sodium levels higher than desired

2005 Electrolyte Management: Hyperphosphatemia
Promotion of phosphate balance and prevention of complications resulting from serum phosphate levels higher than desired

2006 Electrolyte Management: Hypocalcemia
Promotion of calcium balance and prevention of complications resulting from serum calcium levels lower than desired

2007 Electrolyte Management: Hypokalemia
Promotion of potassium balance and prevention of complications resulting from serum potassium levels lower than desired

2008 Electrolyte Management: Hypomagnesemia
Promotion of magnesium balance and prevention of complications resulting from serum magnesium levels lower than desired

2009 Electrolyte Management: Hyponatremia
Promotion of sodium balance and prevention of complications resulting from serum sodium levels lower than desired

2010 Electrolyte Management: Hypophosphatemia
Promotion of phosphate balance and prevention of complications resulting from serum phosphate levels lower than desired

2020 Electrolyte Monitoring
Collection and analysis of patient data to regulate electrolyte balance

6771 Electronic Fetal Monitoring: Antepartum
Electronic evaluation of fetal heart rate response to movement, external stimuli, or uterine contractions during antepartal testing

6772 Electronic Fetal Monitoring: Intrapartum
Electronic evaluation of fetal heart rate response to uterine contractions during intrapartal care

6470 Elopement Precautions
Minimizing the risk of a patient leaving a treatment setting without authorization when departure presents a threat to the safety of patient or others

4104 Embolus Care: Peripheral
Limitation of complications for a patient experiencing, or at risk for, occlusion of peripheral circulation

4106 Embolus Care: Pulmonary
Limitation of complications for a patient experiencing, or at risk for, occlusion of pulmonary circulation

4110 Embolus Precautions
Reduction of the risk of an embolus in a patient with thrombi or at risk for developing thrombus formation

6200 Emergency Care
Providing life-saving measures in life-threatening situations

7660 Emergency Cart Checking
Systematic review of the contents of an emergency cart at established time intervals

5270 Emotional Support
Provision of reassurance, acceptance, and encouragement during times of stress

3270 Endotracheal Extubation
Purposeful removal of the endotracheal tube from the nasopharyngeal or oropharyngeal airway

0180 Energy Management
Regulating energy use to treat or prevent fatigue and optimize function

1056 Enteral Tube Feeding
Delivering nutrients and water through a gastrointestinal tube

6480 Environmental Management
Manipulation of the patient's surroundings for therapeutic benefit

6481 Environmental Management: Attachment Process
Manipulation of the patient's surroundings to facilitate the development of the parent-infant relationship

6482 Environmental Management: Comfort
Manipulation of the patient's surroundings for promotion of optimal comfort

6484 Environmental Management: Community
Monitoring and influencing the direction of the physical, social, cultural, economic, and political conditions that affect the health of groups and communities

6485 Environmental Management: Home Preparation
Preparing the home for safe and effective delivery of care

6486 Environmental Management: Safety
Monitoring and manipulation of the physical environment to promote safety

6487 Environmental Management: Violence Prevention
Monitoring and manipulation of the physical environment to decrease the potential for violent behavior directed toward self, others, or environment

6489 Environmental Management: Worker Safety
Monitoring and manipulating of the worksite environment to promote safety and health of workers

8880 Environmental Risk Protection
Preventing and detecting disease and injury in populations at risk from environmental hazards

7680 Examination Assistance
Providing assistance to the patient and another healthcare provider during a procedure or exam

0200   Exercise Promotion
Facilitation of regular physical exercise to maintain or advance to a higher level of fitness and health

0201   Exercise Promotion: Strength Training
Facilitating regular resistive muscle training to maintain or increase muscle strength

0202   Exercise Promotion: Stretching
Facilitation of systematic slow-stretch-hold muscle exercises to induce relaxation, to prepare muscles/joints for more vigorous exercise, or to increase or maintain body flexibility

0221   Exercise Therapy: Ambulation
Promotion and assistance with walking to maintain or restore autonomic and voluntary body functions during treatment and recovery from illness or injury

0222   Exercise Therapy: Balance
Use of specific activities, postures, and movements to maintain, enhance, or restore balance

0224   Exercise Therapy: Joint Mobility
Use of active or passive body movement to maintain or restore joint flexibility

0226   Exercise Therapy: Muscle Control
Use of specific activity or exercise protocols to enhance or restore controlled body movement

1650   Eye Care
Prevention or minimization of threats to eye or visual integrity

6490   Fall Prevention
Instituting special precautions with patient at risk for injury from falling

7100   Family Integrity Promotion
Promotion of family cohesion and unity

7104   Family Integrity Promotion: Childbearing Family
Facilitation of the growth of individuals or families who are adding an infant to the family unit

7110   Family Involvement Promotion
Facilitating family participation in the emotional and physical care of the patient

7120   Family Mobilization
Utilization of family strengths to influence patient's health in a positive direction

6784   Family Planning: Contraception
Facilitation of pregnancy prevention by providing information about the physiology of reproduction and methods to control conception

6786   Family Planning: Infertility
Management, education, and support of the patient and significant other undergoing evaluation and treatment for infertility

6788   Family Planning: Unplanned Pregnancy
Facilitation of decision-making regarding pregnancy outcome

7130   Family Process Maintenance
Minimization of family process disruption effects

7140   Family Support
Promotion of family values, interests and goals

7150   Family Therapy
Assisting family members to move their family toward a more productive way of living

1050   Feeding
Providing nutritional intake for patient who is unable to feed self

7160   Fertility Preservation
Providing information, counseling, and treatment that facilitate reproductive health and the ability to conceive

3740   Fever Treatment
Management of a patient with hyperpyrexia caused by nonenvironmental factors

7380   Financial Resource Assistance
Assisting an individual/family to secure and manage finances to meet healthcare needs

6500   Fire-Setting Precautions
Prevention of fire setting behaviors

6240   First Aid
Providing initial care of a minor injury

8550   Fiscal Resource Management
Procuring and directing the use of financial resources to assure the development and continuation of programs and services

0470   Flatulence Reduction
Prevention of flatus formation and facilitation of passage of excessive gas

4120   Fluid Management
Promotion of fluid balance and prevention of complications resulting from abnormal or undesired fluid levels

4130   Fluid Monitoring
Collection and analysis of patient data to regulate fluid balance

4140   Fluid Resuscitation
Administering prescribed intravenous fluids rapidly

2080   Fluid/Electrolyte Management
Regulation and prevention of complications from altered fluid and/or electrolyte levels

1660   Foot Care
Cleansing and inspecting the feet for the purposes of relaxation, cleanliness, and healthy skin

5280   Forgiveness Facilitation
Assisting an individual to forgive and/or experience forgiveness in relationship with self, others, and higher power

1080   Gastrointestinal Intubation
Insertion of a tube into the gastrointestinal tract

5242   Genetic Counseling
Use of an interactive helping process focusing on assisting an individual, family, or group, manifesting or at risk for developing or transmitting a birth defect or genetic condition, to cope.

5290   Grief Work Facilitation
Assistance with the resolution of a significant loss

5294   Grief Work Facilitation: Perinatal Death
Assistance with the resolution of a perinatal loss

5300   Guilt Work Facilitation
Helping another to cope with painful feelings of responsibility, actual or perceived

1670   Hair Care
Promotion of neat, clean, attractive hair

6510   Hallucination Management
Promoting the safety, comfort, and reality orientation of a patient experiencing hallucinations

7960   Healthcare Information Exchange
Providing patient care information to health professionals in other agencies

5510   Health Education
Developing and providing instruction and learning experiences to facilitate voluntary adaptation of behavior conducive to health in individuals, families, groups, or communities

7970   Health Policy Monitoring
Surveillance and influence of government and organization regulations, rules, and standards that affect nursing systems and practices to ensure quality care of patients

6520   Health Screening
Detecting health risks or problems by means of history, examination, and other procedures

7400   Health System Guidance
Facilitating a patient's location and use of appropriate health services

3780   Heat Exposure Treatment
Management of patient overcome by heat due to excessive environmental heat exposure

1380   Heat/Cold Application
Stimulation of the skin and underlying tissues with heat or cold for the purpose of decreasing pain, muscle spasms, or inflammation

2100   Hemodialysis Therapy
Management of extracorporeal passage of the patient's blood through a dialyzer

4150   Hemodynamic Regulation
Optimization of heart rate, preload, afterload, and contractility

2110   Hemofiltration Therapy
Cleansing of acutely ill patient's blood via a hemofilter controlled by the patient's hydrostatic pressure

4160   Hemorrhage Control
Reduction or elimination of rapid and excessive blood loss

6800 High-Risk Pregnancy Care
Identification and management of a high-risk pregnancy to promote healthy outcomes for mother and baby

7180 Home Maintenance Assistance
Helping the patient/family to maintain the home as a clean, safe, and pleasant place to live

5310 Hope Instillation
Facilitation of the development of a positive outlook in a given situation

5320 Humor
Facilitating the patient to perceive, appreciate, and express what is funny, amusing, or ludicrous in order to establish relationships, relieve tension, release anger, facilitate learning, or cope with painful feelings

2120 Hyperglycemia Management
Preventing and treating above-normal blood glucose levels

4170 Hypervolemia Management
Reduction in extracellular and/or intracellular fluid volume and prevention of complications in a patient who is fluid overloaded

5920 Hypnosis
Assisting a patient to induce an altered state of consciousness to create an acute awareness and a directed focus experience

2130 Hypoglycemia Management
Preventing and treating low blood glucose levels

3800 Hypothermia Treatment
Rewarming and surveillance of a patient whose core body temperature is below 35° C

4180 Hypovolemia Management
Expansion of intravascular fluid volume in a patient who is volume depleted

6530 Immunization/Vaccination Management
Monitoring immunization status, facilitating access to immunizations, and provision of immunizations to prevent communicable disease

4370 Impulse Control Training
Assisting the patient to mediate impulsive behavior through application of problem-solving strategies to social and interpersonal situations

7980 Incident Reporting
Written and verbal reporting of any event in the process of patient care that is inconsistent with desired patient outcomes or routine operations of the healthcare facility

3440 Incision Site Care
Cleansing, monitoring, and promotion of healing in a wound that is closed with sutures, clips, or staples

6820 Infant Care
Provision of developmentally appropriate family-centered care to the child under 1 year of age

6540 Infection Control
Minimizing the acquisition and transmission of infectious agents

6545 Infection Control: Intraoperative
Preventing nosocomial infection in the operating room

6550 Infection Protection
Prevention and early detection of infection in a patient at risk

7410 Insurance Authorization
Assisting the patient and provider to secure payment for health services or equipment from a third party

2590 Intracranial Pressure (ICP) Monitoring
Measurement and interpretation of patient data to regulate intracranial pressure

6830 Intrapartal Care
Monitoring and management of stages one and two of the birth process

6834 Intrapartal Care: High-Risk Delivery
Assisting vaginal birth of multiple or malpositioned fetuses

4190 Intravenous (IV) Insertion
Insertion of a needle into a peripheral vein for the purpose of administering fluids, blood, or medications

4200 Intravenous (IV) Therapy
Administration and monitoring of intravenous fluids and medications

4210 Invasive Hemodynamic Monitoring
Measurement and interpretation of invasive hemodynamic parameters to determine cardiovascular function and regulate therapy as appropriate

6840 Kangaroo Care
Promoting closeness between parent and physiologically stable preterm infant by preparing the parent and providing the environment for skin-to-skin contact

6850 Labor Induction
Initiation or augmentation of labor by mechanical or pharmacological methods

6860 Labor Suppression
Controlling uterine contractions prior to 37 weeks of gestation to prevent preterm birth

7690 Laboratory Data Interpretation
Critical analysis of patient laboratory data in order to assist with clinical decision-making

5244 Lactation Counseling
Use of an interactive helping process to assist in maintenance of successful breastfeeding

6870 Lactation Suppression
Facilitating the cessation of milk production and minimizing breast engorgement after giving birth

6560 Laser Precautions
Limiting the risk of injury to the patient related to use of a laser

6570   Latex Precautions
Reducing the risk of systemic reaction to latex

5520   Learning Facilitation
Promoting the ability to process and comprehend information

5540   Learning Readiness Enhancement
Improving the ability and willingness to receive information

3460   Leech Therapy
Application of medicinal leeches to help drain replanted or transplanted tissue engorged with venous blood

4380   Limit Setting
Establishing the parameters of desirable and acceptable patient behavior

3840   Malignant Hyperthermia Precautions
Prevention or reduction of hypermetabolic response to pharmacological agents used during surgery

3300   Mechanical Ventilation
Use of an artificial device to assist a patient to breathe

3310   Mechanical Ventilatory Weaning
Assisting the patient to breathe without the aid of a mechanical ventilator

2300   Medication Administration
Preparing, giving, and evaluating the effectiveness of prescription and nonprescription drugs

2308   Medication Administration: Ear
Preparing and instilling otic medications

2301   Medication Administration: Enteral
Delivering medications through an intestinal tube

2309   Medication Administration: Epidural
Preparing and administering medications via the epidural route

2310   Medication Administration: Eye
Preparing and instilling opthalmic medications

2311   Medication Administration: Inhalation
Preparing and administering inhaled medications

2302   Medication Administration: Interpleural
Administration of medication through an interpleural catheter for reduction of pain

2312   Medication Administration: Intradermal
Preparing and giving medications via the intradermal route

2313   Medication Administration: Intramuscular (IM)
Preparing and giving medications via the intramuscular route

2303   Medication Administration: Intraosseous
Insertion of a needle through the bone cortex into the medullary cavity for the purpose of short-term, emergency administration of fluid, blood, or medication

2314   Medication Administration: Intravenous (IV)
Preparing and giving medications via the intravenous route

2304   Medication Administration: Oral
Preparing and giving medications by mouth and monitoring patient responsiveness

2315   Medication Administration: Rectal
Preparing and inserting rectal suppositories

2316   Medication Administration: Skin
Preparing and applying medications to the skin

2317   Medication Administration: Subcutaneous
Preparing and giving medications via the subcutaneous route

2318   Medication Administration: Vaginal
Preparing and inserting vaginal medications

2307   Medication Administration: Ventricular Reservoir
Administration and monitoring of medication through an indwelling catheter into the lateral ventricle

2380   Medication Management
Facilitation of safe and effective use of prescription and over-the-counter drugs

2390   Medication Prescribing
Prescribing medication for a health problem

5960   Meditation Facilitation
Facilitating a person to alter his/her level of awareness by focusing specifically on an image or thought

4760   Memory Training
Facilitation of memory

4390   Milieu Therapy
Use of people, resources, and events in the patient's immediate environment to promote optimal psychosocial functioning

5330   Mood Management
Providing for safety, stabilization, recovery, and maintenance of a patient who is experiencing dysfunctionally depressed mood or elevated mood

8020   Multidisciplinary Care Conference
Planning and evaluating patient care with health professionals from other disciplines

4400   Music Therapy
Using music to help achieve a specific change in behavior, feeling, or physiology

4410   Mutual Goal Setting
Collaborating with patient to identify and prioritize care goals, then developing a plan for achieving those goals

1680   Nail Care
Promotion of clean, neat, attractive nails and prevention of skin lesions related to improper care of nails

1450   Nausea Management
Prevention and alleviation of nausea

2620   Neurologic Monitoring
Collection and analysis of patient data to prevent or minimize neurological complications

6880   Newborn Care
Management of neonate during the transition to extrauterine life and subsequent period of stabilization

6890   Newborn Monitoring
Measurement and interpretation of physiologic status of the neonate the first 24 hours after delivery

6900   Nonnutritive Sucking
Provision of sucking opportunities for the infant

7200   Normalization Promotion
Assisting parents and other family members of children with chronic illnesses or disabilities in providing normal life experiences for their children and families

1100   Nutrition Management
Assisting with or providing a balanced dietary intake of foods and fluids

1120   Nutrition Therapy
Administration of food and fluids to support metabolic processes of a patient who is malnourished or at high risk for becoming malnourished

5246   Nutritional Counseling
Use of an interactive helping process focusing on the need for diet modification

1160   Nutritional Monitoring
Collection and analysis of patient data to prevent or minimize malnourishment

1710   Oral Health Maintenance
Maintenance and promotion of oral hygiene and dental health for the patient at risk for developing oral or dental lesions

1720   Oral Health Promotion
Promotion of oral hygiene and dental care for a patient with normal oral and dental health

1730   Oral Health Restoration
Promotion of healing for a patient who has an oral mucosa or dental lesion

8060   Order Transcription
Transferring information from order sheets to the nursing patient care planning and documentation system

6260   Organ Procurement
Guiding families through the donation process to ensure timely retrieval of vital organs and tissue for transplant

0480   Ostomy Care
Maintenance of elimination through a stoma and care of surrounding tissue

3320   Oxygen Therapy
Administration of oxygen and monitoring of its effectiveness

1400   Pain Management
Alleviation of pain or a reduction in pain to a level of comfort that is acceptable to the patient

5562   Parent Education: Adolescent
Assisting parents to understand and help their adolescent children

5566   Parent Education: Childrearing Family
Assisting parents to understand and promote the physical, psychological, and social growth and development of their toddler, preschool, or school-age child/children

5568   Parent Education: Infant
Instruction on nurturing and physical care needed during the first year of life

8300   Parenting Promotion
Providing parenting information, support, and coordination of comprehensive services to high-risk families

7440   Pass Facilitation
Arranging a leave for a patient from a healthcare facility

4420   Patient Contracting
Negotiating an agreement with a patient that reinforces a specific behavior change

2400   Patient-Controlled Analgesia (PCA) Assistance
Facilitating patient control of analgesic administration and regulation

7460   Patient Rights Protection
Protection of healthcare rights of a patient, especially a minor, an incapacitated, or an incompetent patient unable to make decisions

7700   Peer Review
Systematic evaluation of a peer's performance compared with professional standards of practice

0560   Pelvic Muscle Exercise
Strengthening and training the levator ani and urogenital muscles through voluntary, repetitive contraction to decrease stress, urge, or mixed types of urinary incontinence

1750   Perineal Care
Maintenance of perineal skin integrity and relief of perineal discomfort

2660   Peripheral Sensation Management
Prevention or minimization of injury or discomfort in the patient with altered sensation

4220   Peripherally Inserted Central (PIC) Catheter Care
Insertion and maintenance of a peripherally inserted central catheter

2150   Peritoneal Dialysis Therapy
Administration and monitoring of dialysis solution into and out of the peritoneal cavity

0630   Pessary Management
Placement and monitoring of a vaginal device for treating stress urinary incontinence, uterine retroversion, genital prolapse, or incompetent cervix

4232 Phlebotomy: Arterial Blood Sample
Obtaining a blood sample from an uncannulated artery to assess oxygen and carbon dioxide levels and acid-base balance

4234 Phlebotomy: Blood Unit Acquisition
Procuring blood and blood products from donors

4238 Phlebotomy: Venous Blood Sample
Removal of a sample of venous blood from an uncannulated vein

6924 Phototherapy: Neonate
Use of light therapy to reduce bilirubin levels in newborn infants

6580 Physical Restraint
Application, monitoring, and removal of mechanical restraining devices or manual restraints which are used to limit physical mobility of a patient

7710 Physician Support
Collaborating with physicians to provide quality patient care

6590 Pneumatic Tourniquet Precautions
Applying a pneumatic tourniquet while minimizing the potential for patient injury from use of the device

0840 Positioning
Deliberative placement of the patient or a body part to promote physiological and/or psychological well-being

0842 Positioning: Intraoperative
Moving the patient or body part to promote surgical exposure while reducing the risk of discomfort and complications

0844 Positioning: Neurologic
Achievement of optimal, appropriate body alignment for the patient experiencing or at risk for spinal cord injury or vertebrae irritability

0846 Positioning: Wheelchair
Placement of a patient in a properly selected wheelchair to enhance comfort, promote skin integrity, and foster independence

2870 Postanesthesia Care
Monitoring and management of the patient who has recently undergone general or regional anesthesia

1770 Postmortem Care
Providing physical care of the body of an expired patient and support for the family viewing the body

6930 Postpartal Care
Monitoring and management of the patient who has recently given birth

7722 Preceptor: Employee
Assisting and supporting a new or transferred employee through a planned orientation to a specific clinical area

7726 Preceptor: Student
Assisting and supporting learning experiences for a student

5247 Preconception Counseling
Screening and providing information and support to individuals of childbearing age before pregnancy to promote health and reduce risks

6950 Pregnancy Termination Care
Management of the physical and psychological needs of the woman undergoing a spontaneous or elective abortion

6960 Prenatal Care
Monitoring and management of patient during pregnancy to prevent complications of pregnancy and promote a healthy outcome for both mother and infant

2880 Preoperative Coordination
Facilitating preadmission diagnostic testing and preparation of the surgical patient

5580 Preparatory Sensory Information
Describing in concrete and objective terms the typical sensory experiences and events associated with an upcoming stressful healthcare procedure/treatment

5340 Presence
Being with another, both physically and psychologically, during times of need

3500 Pressure Management
Minimizing pressure to body parts

3520 Pressure Ulcer Care
Facilitation of healing in pressure ulcers

3540 Pressure Ulcer Prevention
Prevention of pressure ulcers for a patient at high risk for developing them

7760 Product Evaluation
Determining the effectiveness of new products or equipment

8700 Program Development
Planning, implementing, and evaluating a coordinated set of activities designed to enhance wellness, or to prevent, reduce, or eliminate one or more health problems or a group or community

1460 Progressive Muscle Relaxation
Facilitating the tensing and releasing of successive muscle groups while attending to the resulting differences in sensation

0640 Prompted Voiding
Promotion of urinary continence through the use of timed verbal toileting reminders and positive social feedback for successful toileting

1780 Prosthesis Care
Care of a removable appliance worn by a patient and prevention of complications associated with its use

3550 Pruritis Management
Preventing and treating itching

7800 Quality Monitoring
Systematic collection and analysis of an organization's quality indicators for the purpose of improving patient care

6600 Radiation Therapy Management
Assisting the patient to understand and minimize the side effects of radiation treatments

6300 Rape-Trauma Treatment
Provision of emotional and physical support immediately following a reported rape

4820 Reality Orientation
Promotion of patient's awareness of personal identity, time, and environment

5360 Recreation Therapy
Purposeful use of recreation to promote relaxation and enhancement of social skills

0490 Rectal Prolapse Management
Prevention and/or manual reduction of rectal prolapse

8100 Referral
Arrangement for services by another care provider or agency

5422 Religious Addiction Prevention
Prevention of a self-imposed controlling religious lifestyle

5424 Religious Ritual Enhancement
Facilitating participation in religious practices

4860 Reminiscence Therapy
Using the recall of past events, feelings, and thoughts to facilitate pleasure, quality of life, or adaptation to present circumstances

7886 Reproductive Technology Management
Assisting a patient through the steps of complex infertility treatment

8120 Research Data Collection
Collecting research data

8340 Resiliency Promotion
Assisting individuals, families, and communities in development, use, and strengthening of protective factors to be used in coping with environmental and societal stressors

3350 Respiratory Monitoring
Collection and analysis of patient data to ensure airway patency and adequate gas exchange

7260 Respite Care
Provision of short-term care to provide relief for family caregiver

6320 Resuscitation
Administering emergency measures to sustain life

6972　Resuscitation: Fetus

Administering emergency measures to improve placental perfusion or correct fetal acid-base status

6974　Resuscitation: Neonate

Administering emergency measures to support newborn adaptation to extrauterine life

6610　Risk Identification

Analysis of potential risk factors, determination of health risks, and prioritization of risk reduction strategies for an individual or group

6612　Risk Identification: Childbearing Family

Identification of an individual or family likely to experience difficulties in parenting and prioritization of strategies to prevent parenting problems

6614　Risk Identification: Genetic

Identification and analysis of potential genetic risk factors in an individual, family, or group

5370　Role Enhancement

Assisting a patient, significant other, and/or family to improve relationships by clarifying and supplementing specific role behaviors

6630　Seclusion

Solitary containment in a fully protective environment with close surveillance by nursing staff for purposes of safety or behavior management

5380　Security Enhancement

Intensifying a patient's sense of physical and psychological safety

2680　Seizure Management

Care of a patient during a seizure and the postictal state

2690　Seizure Precautions

Prevention or minimization of potential injuries sustained by a patient with a known seizure disorder

5390　Self-Awareness Enhancement

Assisting a patient to explore and understand his/her thoughts, feelings, motivations, and behaviors

1800　Self-Care Assistance

Assisting another to perform activities of daily living

1801　Self-Care Assistance: Bathing/Hygiene

Assisting patient to perform personal hygiene

1802　Self-Care Assistance: Dressing/Grooming

Assisting patient with clothes and makeup

1803　Self-Care Assistance: Feeding

Assisting a person to eat

1804　Self-Care Assistance: Toileting

Assisting another with elimination

5400   Self-Esteem Enhancement
Assisting a patient to increase his/her personal judgment of self worth

4470   Self-Modification Assistance
Reinforcement of self-directed change initiated by the patient to achieve personally important goals

4480   Self-Responsibility Facilitation
Encouraging a patient to assume more responsibility for own behavior

5248   Sexual Counseling
Use of an interactive helping process focusing on the need to make adjustments in sexual practice or to enhance coping with a sexual event/disorder

8140   Shift Report
Exchanging essential patient care information with other nursing staff at change of shift

4250   Shock Management
Facilitation of the delivery of oxygen and nutrients to systemic tissue with removal of cellular waste products in a patient with severely altered tissue perfusion

4254   Shock Management: Cardiac
Promotion of adequate tissue perfusion for a patient with severely compromised pumping function of the heart

4256   Shock Management: Vasogenic
Promotion of adequate tissue perfusion for a patient with severe loss of vascular tone

4258   Shock Management: Volume
Promotion of adequate tissue perfusion for a patient with severely compromised intravascular volume

4260   Shock Prevention
Detecting and treating a patient at risk for impending shock

7280   Sibling Support
Assisting a sibling to cope with a brother's or sister's illness/chronic condition/disability

6000   Simple Guided Imagery
Purposeful use of imagination to achieve relaxation and/or direct attention away from undesirable sensations

1480   Simple Massage
Stimulation of the skin and underlying tissues with varying degrees of hand pressure to decrease pain, produce relaxation, and/or improve circulation

6040   Simple Relaxation Therapy
Use of techniques to encourage and elicit relaxation for the purpose of decreasing undesirable signs and symptoms such as pain, muscle tension, or anxiety

3584   Skin Care: Topical Treatments
Application of topical substances or manipulation of devices to promote skin integrity and minimize skin breakdown

3590 Skin Surveillance
Collection and analysis of patient data to maintain skin and mucous membrane integrity

1850 Sleep Enhancement
Facilitation of regular sleep/wake cycles

4490 Smoking Cessation Assistance
Helping another to stop smoking

5100 Socialization Enhancement
Facilitation of another person's ability to interact with others

7820 Specimen Management
Obtaining, preparing, and preserving a specimen for a laboratory test

5426 Spiritual Growth Facilitation
Facilitation of growth in patient's capacity to identify, connect with, and call upon the source of meaning, purpose, comfort, strength, and hope in his/her life

5420 Spiritual Support
Assisting the patient to feel balance and connection with a greater power

0910 Splinting
Stabilization, immobilization, and/or protection of an injured body part with a supportive appliance

6648 Sports-Injury Prevention: Youth
Reduce the risk of sport-related injury in young athletes

7850 Staff Development
Developing, maintaining, and monitoring competence of staff

7830 Staff Supervision
Facilitating the delivery of high-quality patient care by others

2720 Subarachnoid Hemorrhage Precautions
Reduction of internal and external stimuli or stressors to minimize risk of rebleeding prior to aneurysm surgery

4500 Substance Use Prevention
Prevention of an alcoholic or drug use lifestyle

4510 Substance Use Treatment
Supportive care of patient/family members with physical and psychosocial problems associated with the use of alcohol or drugs

4512 Substance Use Treatment: Alcohol Withdrawal
Care of the patient experiencing sudden cessation of alcohol consumption

4514 Substance Use Treatment: Drug Withdrawal
Care of a patient experiencing drug detoxification

4516 Substance Use Treatment: Overdose
Monitoring, treatment, and emotional support of a patient who has ingested prescription or over-the-counter drugs beyond the therapeutic range

6340 Suicide Prevention
Reducing risk of self-inflicted harm with intent to end life

7840 Supply Management
Ensuring acquisition and maintenance of appropriate items for providing patient care

5430 Support Group
Use of a group environment to provide emotional support and health-related information for members

5440 Support System Enhancement
Facilitation of support to patient by family, friends, and community

2900 Surgical Assistance
Assisting the surgeon/dentist with operative procedures and care of the surgical patient

2920 Surgical Precautions
Minimizing the potential for iatrogenic injury to the patient related to a surgical procedure

2930 Surgical Preparation
Providing care to a patient immediately prior to surgery and verification of required procedures/tests and documentation in the clinical record

6650 Surveillance
Purposeful and ongoing acquisition, interpretation, and synthesis of patient data for clinical decision-making

6652 Surveillance: Community
Purposeful and ongoing acquisition, interpretation, and synthesis of data for decision-making in the community

6656 Surveillance: Late Pregnancy
Purposeful and ongoing acquisition, interpretation, and synthesis of maternal-fetal data for treatment, observation, or admission

6658 Surveillance: Remote Electronic
Purposeful and ongoing acquisition of patient data via electronic modalities (telephone, video, conferencing, e-mail) from distant locations as well as interpretation and synthesis of patient data for clinical decision-making with individuals or populations

6654 Surveillance: Safety
Purposeful and ongoing collection and analysis of information about the patient and the environment for use in promoting and maintaining patient safety

7500 Sustenance Support
Helping a needy individual/family to locate food, clothing, or shelter

3620 Suturing
Approximating edges of a wound using sterile suture material and a needle

1860 Swallowing Therapy
Facilitating swallowing and preventing complications of impaired swallowing

5602 Teaching: Disease Process
Assisting the patient to understand information related to a specific disease process

5604   Teaching: Group
Development, implementation, and evaluation of a patient teaching program for a group of individuals experiencing the same health condition

5606   Teaching: Individual
Planning, implementation, and evaluation of a teaching program designed to address a patient's particular needs

5626   Teaching: Infant Nutrition
Instruction on nutrition and feeding practices during the first year of life

5628   Teaching: Infant Safety
Instruction on safety during first year of life

5610   Teaching: Preoperative
Assisting a patient to understand and mentally prepare for surgery and the postoperative recovery period

5612   Teaching: Prescribed Activity/Exercise
Preparing a patient to achieve and/or maintain a prescribed level of activity

5614   Teaching: Prescribed Diet
Preparing a patient to correctly follow a prescribed diet

5616   Teaching: Prescribed Medication
Preparing a patient to safely take prescribed medications and monitor for their effects

5618   Teaching: Procedure/Treatment
Preparing a patient to understand and mentally prepare for a prescribed procedure or treatment

5620   Teaching: Psychomotor Skill
Preparing a patient to perform a psychomotor skill

5622   Teaching: Safe Sex
Providing instruction concerning sexual protection during sexual activity

5624   Teaching: Sexuality
Assisting individuals to understand physical and psychosocial dimensions of sexual growth and development

5630   Teaching: Toddler Nutrition
Instruction on nutrition and feeding practices during the second and third years of life

5632   Teaching: Toddler Safety
Instruction on safety during the second and third years of life

7880   Technology Management
Use of technical equipment and devices to monitor patient condition or sustain life

8180   Telephone Consultation
Eliciting patient's concerns, listening, and providing support, information or teaching in response to patient's stated concerns, over the telephone

8190   Telephone Follow-up
Providing results of testing or evaluating patient's response and determining potential for problems as a result of previous treatment, examination, or testing, over the telephone

3900   Temperature Regulation
Attaining and/or maintaining body temperature within a normal range

3902   Temperature Regulation: Intraoperative
Attaining and/or maintaining desired intraoperative body temperature

4430   Therapeutic Play
Purposeful and directive use of toys and other materials to assist children in communicating their perception and knowledge of their world and to help in gaining mastery of their environment

5465   Therapeutic Touch
Attuning to the universal healing field, seeking to act as an instrument for healing influence, and using the natural sensitivity of the hands to gently focus and direct the intervention process

5450   Therapy Group
Application of psychotherapeutic techniques to a group, including the utilization of interactions between members of the group

1200   Total Parenteral Nutrition (TPN) Administration
Preparation and delivery of nutrients intravenously and monitoring of patient responsiveness

5460   Touch
Providing comfort and communication through purposeful tactile contact

0940   Traction/Immobilization Care
Management of a patient who has traction and/or a stabilizing device to immobilize and stabilize a body part

1540   Transcutaneous Electrical Nerve Stimulation (TENS)
Stimulation of skin and underlying tissues with controlled, low-voltage electrical vibration via electrodes

0960   Transport
Moving a patient from one location to another

6362   Triage: Disaster
Establishing priorities of patient care for urgent treatment while allocating scarce resources

6364   Triage: Emergency Center
Establishing priorities and initiating treatment for patients in an emergency center

6366   Triage: Telephone
Determining the nature and urgency of a problem(s) and providing directions for the level of care required, over the telephone

5470   Truth Telling
Use of whole truth, partial truth, or decision delay to promote the patient's self-determination and well-being

1870 Tube Care
Management of a patient with an external drainage device exiting the body

1872 Tube Care: Chest
Management of a patient with an external water-seal drainage device exiting the chest cavity

1874 Tube Care: Gastrointestinal
Management of a patient with a gastrointestinal tube

1875 Tube Care: Umbilical Line
Management of a newborn with an umbilical catheter

1876 Tube Care: Urinary
Management of a patient with urinary drainage equipment

1878 Tube Care: Ventriculostomy/Lumbar Drain
Management of a patient with an external cerebrospinal fluid drainage system

6982 Ultrasonography: Limited Obstetric
Performance of ultrasound exams to determine ovarian, uterine, or fetal status

2760 Unilateral Neglect Management
Protecting and safely reintegrating the affected part of the body while helping the patient adapt to disturbed perceptual abilities

0570 Urinary Bladder Training
Improving bladder function for those with urge incontinence by increasing the bladder's ability to hold urine and the patient's ability to suppress urination

0580 Urinary Catheterization
Insertion of a catheter into the bladder for temporary or permanent drainage of urine

0582 Urinary Catheterization: Intermittent
Regular periodic use of a catheter to empty the bladder

0590 Urinary Elimination Management
Maintenance of an optimum urinary elimination pattern

0600 Urinary Habit Training
Establishing a predictable pattern of bladder emptying to prevent incontinence for persons with limited cognitive ability who have urge, stress, or functional incontinence

0610 Urinary Incontinence Care
Assistance in promoting continence and maintaining perineal skin integrity

0612 Urinary Incontinence Care: Enuresis
Promotion of urinary continence in children

0620 Urinary Retention Care
Assistance in relieving bladder distention

5480 Values Clarification
Assisting another to clarify her/his own values in order to facilitate effective decision-making

9050   Vehicle Safety Promotion
Assisting individuals, families, and communities to increase awareness of measures to reduce unintentional injuries in motorized and nonmotorized vehicles

2440   Venous Access Devices (VAD) Maintenance
Management of the patient with prolonged venous access via tunneled and nontunneled (percutaneous) catheters and implanted ports

3390   Ventilation Assistance
Promotion of an optimal spontaneous breathing pattern that maximizes oxygen and carbon dioxide exchange in the lungs

7560   Visitation Facilitation
Promoting beneficial visits by family and friends

6680   Vital Signs Monitoring
Collection and analysis of cardiovascular, respiratory, and body temperature data to determine and prevent complications

1570   Vomiting Management
Prevention and alleviation of vomiting

1240   Weight Gain Assistance
Facilitating gain of body weight

1260   Weight Management
Facilitating maintenance of optimal body weight and percent body fat

1280   Weight Reduction Assistance
Facilitating loss of weight and/or body fat

3660   Wound Care
Prevention of wound complications and promotion of wound healing

3662   Wound Care: Closed Drainage
Maintenance of a pressure drainage system at the wound site

3680   Wound Irrigation
Flushing of an open wound to cleanse and remove debris and excessive drainage

NOC Outcome Labels and Definitions
(260 Outcomes)

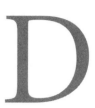

2500 Abuse Cessation
Evidence that the victim is no longer abused

2501 Abuse Protection
Protection of self or dependent others from abuse

2502 Abuse Recovery: Emotional
Healing of psychological injuries due to abuse

2503 Abuse Recovery: Financial
Regaining monetary and legal control or benefits following financial exploitation

2504 Abuse Recovery: Physical
Healing of physical injuries due to abuse

2505 Abuse Recovery: Sexual
Healing following sexual abuse or exploitation

1400 Abusive Behavior Self-Control
Self-restraint of own behaviors to avoid abuse and neglect of dependents or significant others

1300 Acceptance: Health Status
Reconciliation to health circumstances

0005 Activity Tolerance
Responses to energy-consuming body movements involved in required or desired daily activities

1600 Adherence Behavior
Self-initiated action taken to promote wellness, recovery, and rehabilitation

Source: Johnson, M., Maas, M., & Moorhead, S. (2000). *Nursing Outcomes Classification, 2nd ed.* St. Louis: Mosby, Inc. Reproduced with permission of the publisher.

1401   Aggression Control
Self-restraint of assaultive, combative, or destructive behavior toward others

0200   Ambulation: Walking
Ability to walk from place to place

0201   Ambulation: Wheelchair
Ability to move from place to place in a wheelchair

1402   Anxiety Control
Personal actions to eliminate or reduce feelings of apprehension and tension from an unidentifiable source

1918   Aspiration Control
Personal actions to prevent the passage of fluid and solid particles into the lung

0704   Asthma Control
Personal actions to reverse inflammatory condition resulting in bronchial constriction of the airways

0202   Balance
Ability to maintain body equilibrium

2300   Blood Glucose Control
Extent to which plasma glucose levels are maintained in expected range

0700   Blood Transfusion Reaction Control
Extent to which complications of blood transfusions are minimized

1200   Body Image
Positive perception of own appearance and body functions

0203   Body Positioning: Self-Initiated
Ability to change own body positions

1104   Bone Healing
The extent to which cells and tissues have regenerated following bone injury

0500   Bowel Continence
Control of passage of stool from the bowel

0501   Bowel Elimination
Ability of the gastrointestinal tract to form and evacuate stool effectively

1000   Breastfeeding Establishment: Infant
Proper attachment of an infant to and sucking from the mother's breast for nourishment during the first 2 to 3 weeks

1001   Breastfeeding Establishment: Maternal
Maternal establishment of proper attachment of an infant to and sucking from the breast for nourishment during the first 2 to 3 weeks

1002 Breastfeeding Maintenance
Continued nourishment of an infant through breastfeeding

1003 Breastfeeding Weaning
Process leading to the eventual discontinuation of breastfeeding

0400 Cardiac Pump Effectiveness
Extent to which blood is ejected from the left ventricle per minute to support systemic perfusion pressure

2200 Caregiver Adaptation to Patient Institutionalization
Family caregiver adaptation of role when the care recipient is transferred outside the home

2506 Caregiver Emotional Health
Feelings, attitudes, and emotions of a family care provider while caring for a family member or significant other over an extended period of time

2202 Caregiver Home Care Readiness
Preparedness to assume responsibility for the health care of a family member or significant other in the home

2203 Caregiver Lifestyle Disruption
Disturbances in the lifestyle of a family member due to caregiving

2204 Caregiver-Patient Relationship
Positive interactions and connections between the caregiver and care recipient

2205 Caregiver Performance: Direct Care
Provision by family care provider of appropriate personal and health care for a family member or significant other

2206 Caregiver Performance: Indirect Care
Arrangement and oversight of appropriate care for a family member or significant other by family care provider

2507 Caregiver Physical Health
Physical well-being of a family care provider while caring for a family member or significant other over an extended period of time

2208 Caregiver Stressors
The extent of biopsychosocial pressure on a family care provider caring for a family member or significant other over an extended period of time

2508 Caregiver Well-Being
Primary care provider's satisfaction with health and life circumstances

2210 Caregiving Endurance Potential
Factors that promote family care provider continuance over an extended period of time

1301 Child Adaptation to Hospitalization
Child's adaptive response to hospitalization

0100 Child Development: 2 Months
Milestones of physical, cognitive, and psychosocial progression by 2 months of age

0101 Child Development: 4 Months
Milestones of physical, cognitive, and psychosocial progression by 4 months of age

0102 Child Development: 6 Months
Milestones of physical, cognitive, and psychosocial progression by 6 months of age

0103 Child Development: 12 Months
Milestones of physical, cognitive, and psychosocial progression by 12 months of age

0104 Child Development: 2 Years
Milestones of physical, cognitive, and psychosocial progression by 2 years of age

0105 Child Development: 3 Years
Milestones of physical, cognitive, and psychosocial progression by 3 years of age

0106 Child Development: 4 Years
Milestones of physical, cognitive, and psychosocial progression by 4 years of age

0107 Child Development: 5 Years
Milestones of physical, cognitive, and psychosocial progression by 5 years of age

0108 Child Development: Middle Childhood (6-11 Years)
Milestones of physical, cognitive, and psychosocial progression between 6 and 11 years of age

0109 Child Development: Adolescence (12-17 Years)
Milestones of physical, cognitive, and psychosocial progression between 12 and 17 years of age

0401 Circulation Status
Extent to which blood flows unobstructed, unidirectionally, and at an appropriate pressure through large vessels of the systemic and pulmonary circuits

0409 Coagulation Status
Extent to which blood clots within expected period of time

0900 Cognitive Ability
Ability to execute complex mental processes

0901 Cognitive Orientation
Ability to identify person, place, and time

2100 Comfort Level
Feelings of physical and psychological ease

0902 Communication Ability
Ability to receive, interpret, and express spoken, written, and nonverbal messages

0903 Communication: Expressive Ability
Ability to express and interpret verbal and/or nonverbal messages

0904 Communication: Receptive Ability
Ability to receive and interpret verbal and/or nonverbal messages

2700 Community Competence
The ability of a community to collectively problem-solve to achieve goals

2701 Community Health Status
The general state of well-being of a community or population

2800 Community Health: Immunity
Resistance of a group to the invasion and spread of an infectious agent

2801 Community Risk Control: Chronic Disease
Community actions to reduce the risk of chronic diseases and related complications

2802 Community Risk Control: Communicable Disease
Community actions to eliminate or reduce the spread of infectious agents (bacteria, fungi, parasites, and viruses) that threaten public health

2803 Community Risk Control: Lead Exposure
Community actions to reduce lead exposure and poisoning

1601 Compliance Behavior
Actions taken on the basis of professional advice to promote wellness, recovery, and rehabilitation

0905 Concentration
Ability to focus on a specific stimulus

1302 Coping
Actions to manage stressors that tax an individual's resources

0906 Decision-Making
Ability to choose between two or more alternatives

1409 Depression Control
Personal actions to minimize melancholy and maintain interest in life events

1208 Depression Level
Severity of melancholic mood and loss of interest in life events

1105 Dialysis Access Integrity
The extent to which a dialysis access site is functional and free of inflammation

1303 Dignified Dying
Maintaining personal control and comfort with the approaching end of life

1403 Distorted Thought Control
Self-restraint of disruption in perception, thought processes, and thought content

0600 Electrolyte & Acid/Base Balance
Balance of the electrolytes and nonelectrolytes in the intracellular and extracellular compartments of the body

0001 Endurance
Extent that energy enables a person to sustain activity

0002 Energy Conservation
Extent of active management of energy to initiate and sustain activity

2600 Family Coping
Family actions to manage stressors that tax family resources

2601 Family Environment: Internal
Social climate as characterized by family member relationships and goals

2602 Family Functioning
Ability of the family to meet the needs of its members through developmental transitions

2606 Family Health Status
Overall health status and social competence of family unit

2603 Family Integrity
Extent that family members' behaviors collectively demonstrate cohesion, strength, and emotional bonding

2604 Family Normalization
Ability of the family to develop and maintain routines and management strategies that contribute to optimal functioning when a member has a chronic illness or disability

2605 Family Participation in Professional Care
Family involvement in decision-making, delivery, and evaluation of care provided by healthcare personnel

1404 Fear Control
Personal actions to eliminate or reduce disabling feelings of alarm aroused by an identifiable source

0111 Fetal Status: Antepartum
Conditions indicative of fetal physical well-being from conception to the onset of labor

0112 Fetal Status: Intrapartum
Conditions and behaviors indicative of fetal well-being from onset of labor to delivery

0601 Fluid Balance
Balance of water in the intracellular and extracellular compartments of the body

1304 Grief Resolution
Adjustment to actual or impending loss

0110 Growth
A normal increase in body size and weight

1700 Health Beliefs
Personal convictions that influence health behaviors

1701 Health Beliefs: Perceived Ability to Perform
Personal conviction that one can carry out a given health behavior

1702 Health Beliefs: Perceived Control
Personal conviction that one can influence a health outcome

1703 Health Beliefs: Perceived Resources
Personal conviction that one has adequate means to carry out a health behavior

1704 Health Beliefs: Perceived Threat
Personal conviction that a health problem is serious and has potential negative consequences for lifestyle

1705 Health Orientation
Personal view of health and health behaviors as priorities

1602 Health Promoting Behavior
Actions to sustain or increase wellness

1603 Health Seeking Behavior
Actions to promote optimal wellness, recovery, and rehabilitation

1610 Hearing Compensation Behavior
Actions to identify, monitor, and compensate for hearing loss

1201 Hope
Presence of internal state of optimism that is personally satisfying and life-supporting

0602 Hydration
Amount of water in the intracellular and extracellular compartments of the body

1202 Identity
Ability to distinguish between self and nonself and to characterize one's essence

0204 Immobility Consequences: Physiological
Extent of compromise in physiological functioning due to impaired physical mobility

0205 Immobility Consequences: Psycho-Cognitive
Extent of compromise in psycho-cognitive functioning due to impaired physical mobility

0701 Immune Hypersensitivity Control
Extent to which inappropriate immune responses are suppressed

0702 Immune Status
Adequacy of natural and acquired appropriately targeted resistance to internal and external antigens

1900 Immunization Behavior
Actions to obtain immunization to prevent a communicable disease

1405 Impulse Control
Self-restraint of compulsive or impulsive behaviors

0703 Infection Status
Presence and extent of infection

0907 Information Processing
Ability to acquire, organize, and use information

0206 Joint Movement: Active
Range of motion of joints with self-initiated movement

0207 Joint Movement: Passive
Range of motion of joints with assisted movement

1800 Knowledge: Breastfeeding
Extent of understanding conveyed about lactation and nourishment of infant through breastfeeding

1801 Knowledge: Child Safety
Extent of understanding conveyed about safely caring for a child

1821 Knowledge: Conception Prevention
Extent of understanding conveyed about pregnancy prevention

1820 Knowledge: Diabetes Management
Extent of understanding conveyed about diabetes mellitus and its control

1802 Knowledge: Diet
Extent of understanding conveyed about diet

1803 Knowledge: Disease Process
Extent of understanding conveyed about a specific disease process

1804 Knowledge: Energy Conservation
Extent of understanding conveyed about energy conservation techniques

1816 Knowledge: Fertility Promotion
Extent of understanding conveyed about fertility testing and the conditions that affect conception

1805 Knowledge: Health Behaviors
Extent of understanding conveyed about the promotion and protection of health

1823 Knowledge: Health Promotion
Extent of understanding of information needed to obtain and maintain optimal health

1806 Knowledge: Health Resources
Extent of understanding conveyed about healthcare resources

1824 Knowledge: Illness Care
Extent of understanding of illness-related information needed to achieve and maintain optimal health

1819 Knowledge: Infant Care
Extent of understanding conveyed about caring for a baby up to 12 months

1807 Knowledge: Infection Control
Extent of understanding conveyed about prevention and control of infection

1817 Knowledge: Labor and Delivery
Extent of understanding conveyed about labor and delivery

1825 Knowledge: Maternal-Child Health
Extent of understanding of information needed to achieve and maintain optimal health of a mother and child

1808   Knowledge: Medication
Extent of understanding conveyed about the safe use of medication

1809   Knowledge: Personal Safety
Extent of understanding conveyed about preventing unintentional injuries

1818   Knowledge: Postpartum
Extent of understanding conveyed about maternal health following delivery

1822   Knowledge: Preconception
Extent of understanding conveyed about maternal health prior to conception to insure a
healthy pregnancy

1810   Knowledge: Pregnancy
Extent of understanding conveyed about maintenance of a healthy pregnancy and
prevention of complications

1811   Knowledge: Prescribed Activity
Extent of understanding conveyed about prescribed activity and exercise

1815   Knowledge: Sexual Functioning
Extent of understanding conveyed about sexual development and responsible sexual
practices

1812   Knowledge: Substance Use Control
Extent of understanding conveyed about managing substance use safely

1814   Knowledge: Treatment Procedure(s)
Extent of understanding conveyed about procedure(s) required as part of a treatment
regimen

1813   Knowledge: Treatment Regimen
Extent of understanding conveyed about a specific treatment regimen

1604   Leisure Participation
Use of restful or relaxing activities as needed to promote well-being

1203   Loneliness
The extent of emotional, social, or existential isolation response

2509   Maternal Status: Antepartum
Conditions and behaviors indicative of maternal well-being from conception to the onset
of labor

2510   Maternal Status: Intrapartum
Conditions and behaviors indicative of maternal well-being from onset of labor to delivery

2511   Maternal Status: Postpartum
Conditions and behaviors indicative of maternal well-being from delivery of placenta to
completion of involution

2301 Medication Response
Therapeutic and adverse effects of prescribed medication

0908 Memory
Ability to cognitively retrieve and report previously stored information

0208 Mobility Level
Ability to move purposefully

1204 Mood Equilibrium
Appropriate adjustment of prevailing emotional tone in response to circumstances

0209 Muscle Function
Adequacy of muscle contraction needed for movement

2512 Neglect Recovery
Healing following the cessation of substandard care

0909 Neurological Status
Extent to which the peripheral and central nervous systems receive, process, and respond to internal and external stimuli

0910 Neurological Status: Autonomic
Extent to which the autonomic nervous system coordinates visceral function

0911 Neurological Status: Central Motor Control
Extent to which skeletal muscle activity (body movement) is coordinated by the central nervous system

0912 Neurological Status: Consciousness
Extent to which an individual arouses, orients, and attends to the environment

0913 Neurological Status: Cranial Sensory/Motor Function
Extent to which cranial nerves convey sensory and motor information

0914 Neurological Status: Spinal Sensory/Motor Function
Extent to which spinal nerves convey sensory and motor information

0118 Newborn Adaptation
Adaptation to the extrauterine environment by a physiologically mature newborn during the first 28 days

1004 Nutritional Status
Extent to which nutrients are available to meet metabolic needs

1005 Nutritional Status: Biochemical Measures
Body fluid components and chemical indices of nutritional status

1006 Nutritional Status: Body Mass
Congruence of body weight, muscle, and fat to height, frame, and gender

1007 Nutritional Status: Energy
Extent to which nutrients provide cellular energy

1008 Nutritional Status: Food & Fluid Intake
Amount of food and fluid taken into the body over a 24-hour period

1009   Nutritional Status: Nutrient Intake
Adequacy of nutrients taken into the body

1100   Oral Health
Condition of the mouth, teeth, gums, and tongue

1605   Pain Control
Personal actions to control pain

2101   Pain: Disruptive Effects
Observed or reported disruptive effects of pain on emotions and behavior

2102   Pain Level
Severity of reported or demonstrated pain

1306   Pain: Psychological Response
Cognitive and emotional responses to physical pain

1500   Parent-Infant Attachment
Behaviors that demonstrate an enduring affectionate bond between a parent and infant

2211   Parenting
Provision of an environment that promotes optimum growth and development of dependent children

1901   Parenting: Social Safety
Parental actions to avoid social relationships that might cause harm or injury

1606   Participation: Health Care Decisions
Personal involvement in selecting and evaluating healthcare options

0113   Physical Aging Status
Physical changes that commonly occur with adult aging

2004   Physical Fitness
Ability to perform physical activities with vigor

0114   Physical Maturation: Female
Normal physical changes in the female that occur with the transition from childhood to adulthood

0115   Physical Maturation: Male
Normal physical changes in the male that occur with the transition from childhood to adulthood

0116   Play Participation

Use of activities as needed for enjoyment, entertainment, and development by children

1607   Prenatal Health Behavior
Personal actions to promote a healthy pregnancy

0117   Preterm Infant Organization
Extrauterine integration of physiologic and behavioral function by the infant born at 24 to 37 (term) weeks gestation

0006   Psychomotor Energy
Ability to maintain activities of daily living (ADL), nutrition and personal safety

1305   Psychosocial Adjustment: Life Change
Psychosocial adaptation of an individual to a life change

2000   Quality of Life
An individual's expressed satisfaction with current life circumstances

0410   Respiratory Status: Airway Patency
Extent to which the tracheobronchial passages remain open

0402   Respiratory Status: Gas Exchange
Alveolar exchange of CO_2 or O_2 to maintain arterial blood gas concentrations

0403   Respiratory Status: Ventilation
Movement of air in and out of the lungs

0003   Rest
Extent and pattern of diminished activity for mental and physical rejuvenation

1902   Risk Control
Actions to eliminate or reduce actual, personal, and modifiable health threats

1903   Risk Control: Alcohol Use
Actions to eliminate or reduce alcohol use that poses a threat to health

1917   Risk Control: Cancer
Actions to reduce or detect the possibility of cancer

1914   Risk Control: Cardiovascular Health
Actions to eliminate or reduce threats to cardiovascular health

1904   Risk Control: Drug Use
Actions to eliminate or reduce drug use that poses a threat to health

1915   Risk Control: Hearing Impairment
Actions to eliminate or reduce the possibility of altered hearing function

1905   Risk Control: Sexually Transmitted Diseases (STD)
Actions to eliminate or reduce behaviors associated with sexually transmitted disease

1906   Risk Control: Tobacco Use
Actions to eliminate or reduce tobacco use

1907   Risk Control: Unintended Pregnancy
Actions to reduce the possibility of unintended pregnancy

1916   Risk Control: Visual Impairment
Actions to eliminate or reduce the possibility of altered visual function

1908   Risk Detection
Actions taken to identify personal health threats

1501   Role Performance
Congruence of an individual's role behavior with role expectations

1909 Safety Behavior: Fall Prevention
Individual or caregiver actions to minimize risk factors that might precipitate falls

1910 Safety Behavior: Home Physical Environment
Individual or caregiver actions to minimize environmental factors that might cause physical harm or injury in the home

1911 Safety Behavior: Personal
Individual or caregiver efforts to control behaviors that might cause physical injury

1912 Safety Status: Falls Occurrence
Number of falls in the past week

1913 Safety Status: Physical Injury
Severity of injuries from accidents and trauma

0300 Self-Care: Activities of Daily Living (ADL)
Ability to perform the most basic physical tasks and personal care activities

0301 Self-Care: Bathing
Ability to cleanse own body

0302 Self-Care: Dressing
Ability to dress self

0303 Self-Care: Eating
Ability to prepare and ingest food

0304 Self-Care: Grooming
Ability to maintain kempt appearance

0305 Self-Care: Hygiene
Ability to maintain own hygiene

0306 Self-Care: Instrumental Activities of Daily Living (IADL)
Ability to perform activities needed to function in the home or community

0307 Self-Care: Non-Parenteral Medication
Ability to administer oral and topical medications to meet therapeutic goals

0308 Self-Care: Oral Hygiene
Ability to care for own mouth and teeth

0309 Self-Care: Parenteral Medication
Ability to administer parenteral medications to meet therapeutic goals

0310 Self-Care: Toileting
Ability to toilet self

1613 Self-Direction of Care
Directing others to assist with or perform physical tasks, personal care, and activities needed to function in the home or the community

1205   Self-Esteem
Personal judgment of self-worth

1406   Self-Mutilation Restraint
Ability to refrain from intentional self-inflicted injury (nonlethal)

2400   Sensory Function: Cutaneous
Extent to which stimulation of the skin is sensed in an impaired area

2401   Sensory Function: Hearing
Extent to which sounds are sensed, with or without assistive devices

2402   Sensory Function: Proprioception
Extent to which the position and movement of the head and body are sensed

2403   Sensory Function: Taste & Smell
Extent to which chemicals inhaled or dissolved in saliva are sensed

2404   Sensory Function: Vision
Extent to which visual images are sensed, with or without assistive devices

0119   Sexual Functioning
Integration of physical, socioemotional, and intellectual aspects of sexual expression

1207   Sexual Identity: Acceptance
Acknowledgment and acceptance of own sexual identity

0211   Skeletal Function
The functional ability of the bones to support the body and facilitate movement

0004   Sleep
Extent and pattern of natural periodic suspension of consciousness during which the body is restored

1502   Social Interaction Skills
An individual's use of effective interaction behaviors

1503   Social Involvement
Frequency of an individual's social interactions with persons, groups, or organizations

1504   Social Support
Perceived availability and actual provision of reliable assistance from other persons

2001   Spiritual Well-Being
Personal expressions of connectedness with self, others, higher power, all life, nature, and the universe that transcend and empower the self

1407   Substance Addiction Consequences
Compromise in health status and social functioning due to substance addiction

2003   Suffering Level
Severity of anguish associated with a distressing symptom, injury, or loss with potential long-term effects

1408   Suicide Self-Restraint
Ability to refrain from gestures and attempts at killing self

1010   Swallowing Status
Extent of safe passage of fluids and/or solids from the mouth to the stomach

1011   Swallowing Status: Esophageal Phase
Adequacy of the passage of fluids and/or solids from the pharynx to the stomach

1012   Swallowing Status: Oral Phase
Adequacy of preparation, containment, and posterior movement of fluids and/or solids in the mouth for swallowing

1013   Swallowing Status: Pharyngeal Phase
Adequacy of the passage of fluids and/or solids from the mouth to the esophagus

1608   Symptom Control
Personal actions to minimize perceived adverse changes in physical and emotional functioning

2103   Symptom Severity
Extent of perceived adverse changes in physical, emotional, and social functioning

2104   Symptom Severity: Perimenopause
Extent of symptoms caused by declining hormonal levels

2105   Symptom Severity: Premenstrual Syndrome (PMS)
Extent of symptoms caused by cyclic hormonal fluctuations

2302   Systemic Toxin Clearance: Dialysis
Extent to which toxins are cleared from the body with peritoneal or hemodialysis

0800   Thermoregulation
Balance among heat production, heat gain, and heat loss

0801   Thermoregulation: Neonate

Balance among heat production, heat gain, and heat loss during the neonatal period

1101   Tissue Integrity: Skin & Mucous Membranes
Structural intactness and normal physiological function of skin and mucous membranes

0404   Tissue Perfusion: Abdominal Organs
Extent to which blood flows through the small vessels of the abdominal viscera and maintains organ function

0405   Tissue Perfusion: Cardiac
Extent to which blood flows through the coronary vasculature and maintains heart function

0406   Tissue Perfusion: Cerebral
Extent to which blood flows through the cerebral vasculature and maintains brain function

0407   Tissue Perfusion: Peripheral
Extent to which blood flows through the small vessels of the extremities and maintains tissue function

0408   Tissue Perfusion: Pulmonary
Extent to which blood flows through intact pulmonary vasculature with appropriate pressure and volume, perfusing alveoli/capillary unit

0210   Transfer Performance
Ability to change body locations

1609   Treatment Behavior: Illness or Injury
Personal actions to palliate or eliminate pathology

0502   Urinary Continence
Control of the elimination of urine

0503   Urinary Elimination
Ability of the urinary system to filter wastes, conserve solutes, and collect and discharge urine in a healthy pattern

1611   Vision Compensation Behavior
Actions to compensate for visual impairment

0802   Vital Signs Status
Temperature, pulse, respiration, and blood pressure within expected range for the individual

1612   Weight Control
Personal actions resulting in achievement and maintenance of optimum body weight for health

2002   Well-Being
An individual's expressed satisfaction with health status

1206   Will to Live
Desire, determination, and effort to survive

1102   Wound Healing: Primary Intention
The extent to which cells and tissues have regenerated following intentional closure

1103   Wound Healing: Secondary Intention
The extent to which cells and tissues in an open wound have regenerated

Timeline and Highlights in Language Development: NANDA, NIC, and NOC

E

1973

▌ Kristine Gebbie and Mary Ann Lavin call the first National Conference for Classification of Nursing Diagnoses at St. Louis, Missouri. A task force is established to carry on the work, and Marjory Gordon is appointed chairperson of the task force, serving in this position during 1973–1982.

▌ A Clearinghouse for Nursing Diagnoses is established at St. Louis University and serves as a repository for information on nursing diagnosis, publishes a newsletter, coordinates plans for national conferences, and distributes bibliographies on each diagnostic category.

1974–2002

▌ Kristine Gebbie and Mary Ann Lavin publish the *First Conference Proceedings*. Conference proceedings have been published following every national conference since that time. Nursecom will publish the most recent proceedings in 2002–2003. Rosemary Carroll-Johnson, Mary Hurley, Mi Ja Kim, Pricilla LeMone, Gertrude McFarland, Audrey McLane, Derry Moritz, Mary Paquette, and Marilyn Rantz have served as editors of the *Proceedings*.

1977–1980

▌ Sr. Callista Roy facilitates the nurse theorist group (i.e., Martha Rogers, Margaret Newman, Dorothea Orem, Imogene King, and others) to develop a framework for organizing nursing diagnoses. The resulting framework, *Patterns of Unitary Man (humans)*, is presented in 1982 to conference participants and is accepted by the membership as the organizing framework for nursing diagnoses.

1982

▌ The North American Nursing Diagnosis Association (NANDA) is formed, incorporating the National Task Force developed to Name and Classify Nursing Diagnoses. Marjory Gordon is elected first president and serves until 1993. Subsequent presidents include Jane Lancour, Lois Hoskins, Judy Warren, Dorothy Jones, Kay Avant, and Mary Anne Lavin.

1982

▌ The American Nurses Association establishes a steering Committee on Classification of Nursing Phenomena, and NANDA's president becomes a committee member.

1985

▌ The Nursing Minimum Data Set Conference includes nursing diagnoses, interventions, and outcomes as key elements in the minimum data set; Springer presents publication of the Nursing Minimum Data Set book by Werley and Lang in 1988.

1986

▌ The American Nurses Association forwards NANDA's Classification of Nursing Diagnosis to the World Health Association for possible inclusion as a chapter in the next edition of the International Classification of Disease (ICD).

1987

▌ NANDA and the American Nurses Association (ANA) develop a model to collaborate on the development of nursing diagnoses.
▌ NANDA publishes Taxonomy 1, with NANDA-approved nursing diagnoses organized under the nine patterns within the framework of *Patterns of Unitary Man (humans)*. Phyllis Kritick serves as first chairperson of the Taxonomy Committee.
▌ The nursing intervention research team is formed at the University of Iowa.

1989

▌ NANDA holds an International Invitational Research Conference on nursing diagnoses, research methodologies, and nursing diagnoses development in Palm Springs, California, facilitated by Gertrude McFarland.

1990

▌ J. B. Lippincott publishes *Nursing Diagnosis*, the official NANDA journal. Rosemary Carroll-Johnson is the journal's first and current editor.
▌ NANDA is included in the Cumulative Index to Nursing and Health Care Literature (CINAHL) and is added to the National Library of Medicine's Methathesaurus for a Unified Medical Language.
▌ The Iowa research team led by Joanne McCloskey and Gloria Bulechek is funded by a research grant from NINR (1990–1993).
▌ The first publication about Nursing Interventions Classification (NIC) appears in print in the *Journal of Professional Nursing*

1991

- The American Nurses Association recognizes *Nursing Interventions Classification* (NIC).
- The Nursing Outcomes research team is formed at the University of Iowa.

1992

- *Nursing Interventions Classification (NIC), 1st edition*, is published by Mosby.
- The Nursing Outcomes Classification (NOC) pilot work is funded by Sigma Theta Tau International, with Marion Johnson and Meridian Maas as the principal investigators.

1993

- NIC is added to National Library of Medicine's Methathesaurus for a Unified Medical Language.
- The second NIC intervention grant is funded by NINR (June 1993–1997 and extended to 1998), with Joanne McCloskey and Gloria Bulechek as the co-principal investigators.
- NOC is funded by NINR (December 1993–1997, extended to 1998), with Marion Johnson and Meridean Maas as the co-principal investigators.
- NANDA and NIC are included in the International Council of Nurses (ICN) *International Classification for Nursing Practice (Alpha version).*
- *The NIC Newsletter* is begun (later changed to *The NIC/NOC Letter*) at the University of Iowa.
- Nursecom becomes the business manager for NANDA membership, with the NANDA Board of Directors maintaining control over organizational director, finances, and activities. Licensing agreements are established with vendors.
- *NANDA: Definitions and Classification* is translated into several languages, including French, Spanish, Portuguese, Dutch, and Japanese.

1994

- Cumulative Index to Nursing and Health Care Literature (CINAHL) and Silver Platter add NIC to their indexes.
- The Joint Commission on Accreditation of Health Care Organizations (JCAHO) includes NIC as a means to meet the standard on uniform data collection.
- The National League for Nursing makes a video describing the work of NIC.
- An institutional effectiveness grant for preparing pre- and postdoctoral students is funded at Iowa (Joanne McCloskey and Meridean Maas, Directors).
- The Nursing Classifications Fund to provide ongoing financial support for the continued development and use of NIC and NOC is established at the University of Iowa.
- NANDA signs a collaborative agreement with a research team at the University of Iowa, NDEC (Nursing Diagnosis and Extension Classification), led by Martha Craft-Rosenberg, Connie Delaney (and, later, Janice Denehy), to improve the scope and clinical usefulness of the NANDA taxonomy.

1995

- The NANDA Foundation is developed to support research on the nursing diagnoses. Currently, a board of directors oversees the Foundation and works to fund nursing diagnosis research on a regular basis.
- The first publication about the *Nursing Outcomes Classification (*NOC) appears in print.
- The Center for Nursing Classification at the University of Iowa is approved (December 13) by the Iowa Board of Regents (without funding) to facilitate the ongoing research and implementation of NIC and NOC. A fundraising advisory board for the Center is established and members are appointed.

1996

- Mosby publishes *Nursing Interventions Classification, 2nd edition*.
- The first meeting of the Center's Fundraising Advisory Board is held.
- The ANA's *Social Policy Statement* includes the NIC definition of an intervention.
- The first vendor (ERGO) signs a licensing agreement for NIC and NOC.
- NIC is linked to the Omaha classification and is distributed in a monograph published by the Center.

1997

- The NANDA journal title is changed to *Nursing Diagnosis: The Journal of Nursing Language and Classification* to encourage the inclusion of other languages in the publication.
- The first joint international NANDA, NIC, NOC Conference is held in St. Charles, Illinois.
- The *Nursing Outcomes Classification (NOC), 1st edition*, is published by Mosby.
- The *NIC Letter* becomes *The NIC/NOC Letter*.

1998

- The second outcomes research grant is funded by NINR (1998–2002) with three PIs: Marion Johnson, Meridean Maas, and Sue Moorhead.
- NANDA, NOC is recognized by the American Nurses Association.
- The Cumulative Index to Nursing and Health Care Literature (CINAHL) adds NOC to their index.
- NIC and NOC submit information to ANSI HISB (American National Standards Institute Health Informatics Standards Board) for Inventory of Clinical Information Standards.
- Mosby YearBook sponsors *The NIC/NOC Letter*.
- Multiple translations of NIC and NOC are processed (Dutch, Korean, Chinese, French, Japanese, German, Spanish), representing the international interest in the classifications.
- The Center for Nursing Classification receives three years of support from the College of Nursing (1998–2001) and is given space on the fourth floor of the College of Nursing; Joanne McCloskey is appointed director.

- NOC is added to National Library of Medicine's Metathesaurus.
- The 1998 NANDA conference in St. Louis, Missouri, celebrates NANDA's twenty-fifth anniversary. The Gebbie and Lavin "Founders Awards" are established. The Proceedings of this conference include over 150 pages documenting the work of NDEC, including the revision or addition of 96 diagnoses.
- The NANDA Archives are established at Boston College, Burns Library, in Boston, Massachusetts.

1999

- NIC is included in Alternative Link *ABC Codes* for reimbursement.
- The first Institute on Informatics and Classification is held in Iowa City, Iowa.
- The NANDA web site is developed (www.nanda.org).
- NANDA, NIC, and NOC, along with other nursing language developers, give testimony about each language classification to a subcommittee of the National Committee on Vital and Health Statistics (NCHVS). The goal is to include nursing language into the standardized Patient Medical Record Information (PMRI).
- NANDA, NIC, and NOC representatives participate in an invitational vocabulary conference at Vanderbilt University in Nashville, directed by Judy Osbolt, with a goal toward developing a reference terminology for nursing.
- NANDA, NIC, and NOC representatives attend an invitational meeting of the SNOMED (Systematized Nomenclature of Medicine) Convergent terminology group in Chicago, Illinois.
- A second joint NANDA, NIC, and NOC conference is held in New Orleans, Louisiana.

2000

- The *Nursing Interventions Classification, 3rd edition*, and the *Nursing Outcomes Classification, 2nd edition*, are published.
- The NNN (3N) Alliance is created as a virtual organization in order to foster a working relationship between NANDA, NIC, and NOC, with Joanne McCloskey Dochterman and Dorothy Jones serving as co-chairs of the Alliance, along with a governing board, including members of the NANDA Board and Center for Nursing Classification Board at Iowa.
- NIC and NOC are linked with the Long Term Care Minimum Data Set Resident Assessment Instrument's (RAI) Resident Assessment Protocols (RAPs) and with OASIS (Outcome and Assessment Information Set) and published in two monographs.
- NOC is linked to the Omaha classification.

2001

- The organizing framework for the NANDA Classification of Nursing Diagnosis is revised; Taxonomy 2 is published with 13 domains and 26 classes plus 7 axes.
- NANDA members vote to change the name of the organization from NANDA to NANDA International to reflect the growing international membership and interest.

- The book that links the three languages—*Nursing Diagnoses, Outcomes, Interventions: NANDA, NOC, and NIC Linkages*—is authored by the NIC and NOC PIs and is published by Mosby.
- A NNN Invitational Common Structure Conference is funded by the National Library of Medicine (Joanne Dochterman and Dorothy Jones, PIs) and is held in Utica, Illinois, in August.
- An effectiveness grant is funded (NINR and AHRQ) for large database research using NIC (Marita Titler and Joanne Dochterman). This is likely the first such grant to fund nursing effectiveness research using a clinical database with nursing standardized language.
- The Center for Nursing Classification receives three years of support from the University of Iowa's central administrative offices.
- NANDA, NIC, and NOC are registered in HL7 (Health Level 7).
- Margaret Lunney edits *Critical Thinking and Nursing Diagnosis: Case Studies and Analysis,* published by Nurscom, with proceeds donated to the NANDA Foundation for research and development.

2002

- The NNN Alliance holds an international conference on nursing language, classification, and informatics in Chicago, Illinois. NANDA's biennial conference becomes integrated into the 3N meeting. A *White Paper on the Development of a Common Structure for NANDA, NIC, and NOC* (forerunner of this publication*)* is presented to participants.
- *SNOMED* (Systematized Nomenclature of Medicine) licenses NANDA, NIC, and NOC for inclusion into their database.
- The Center for Nursing Classification expands its name to the Center for Nursing Classification and Clinical Effectiveness; its endowment reaches $600,000.
- A four-hour web course on standardized languages, NANDA, NIC, and NOC, is offered by the Center for Nursing Classification and Clinical Effectiveness at the University of Iowa.
- A second T-32 training grant for training pre- and postdoctoral students in effectiveness research is funded at Iowa by NINR (with Joanne Dochterman and Martha Craft-Rosenberg as directors).
- The position of Fellow, Center for Nursing Classification and Clinical Effectiveness, is established (to assist in the ongoing development of NIC and NOC), and about 30 people are appointed for three-year terms.

2003

- NANDA, NIC, NOC software program based on linkage book is produced by Mosby.
- NANDA, NIC and NOC continue to develop their respective classifications and, in addition, work to incorporate languages into the proposed NNN Common Structure.

Index

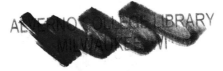